Preparing for Professional Practice in Health and Social Care

Edited by

Anita Atwal
Lecturer in Occupational Therapy, Brunel University, and Director of the Centre for Professional Practice Research

and

Mandy Jones
Lecturer in Physiotherapy, Brunel University

WILEY-BLACKWELL

A John Wiley & Sons, Ltd., Publication

Blackwell Publishing was acquired by John Wiley & Sons in February 2007. Blackwell's publishing programme has been merged with Wiley's global Scientific, Technical, and Medical business to form Wiley-Blackwell.

Registered office
John Wiley & Sons Ltd, The Atrium, Southern Gate, Chichester, West Sussex, PO19 8SQ, United Kingdom

Editorial offices
9600 Garsington Road, Oxford, OX4 2DQ, United Kingdom
2121 State Avenue, Ames, Iowa 50014-8300, USA

For details of our global editorial offices, for customer services and for information about how to apply for permission to reuse the copyright material in this book please see our website at www.wiley.com/wiley-blackwell.

Library of Congress Cataloging-in-Publication Data

Preparing for professional practice in health and social care/[edited] by Anita Atwal and Mandy Jones.
    p. ; cm.
  Includes bibliographical references and index.
  ISBN 978-1-4051-7593-7 (pbk. : alk. paper) 1. Occupational therapy–Practice. 2. Physical therapy–
Practice. I. Atwal, Anita. II. Jones, M. (Mandy), 1967–
  [DNLM: 1. Allied Health Occupations. 2. Allied Health Personnel. 3. Interprofessional Relations. 4. Professional Practice. 5. Professional-Patient Relations. W 21.5 P927 2009]

  RM735.4.P74 2009
  615.8'515–dc22

               2008052867

A catalogue record for this book is available from the British Library.

Set in 10/12 Palatino by Macmillan Publishing Solutions, Chennai, India (www.macmillansolutions.com)
Printed in Singapore by Markono Print Media Pte Ltd

1 2009

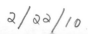
2/22/10

Contents

Contributors list

Introduction:

Shari Rone-Adams
Lecturer in Physiotherapy
School of Health Sciences and
    Social Care
Brunel University
Mary Seacole Building
Uxbridge
Middlesex UB8 3PH

Alex Harvey
Lecturer in Physiotherapy
School of Health Sciences and
    Social Care
Brunel University
Mary Seacole Building
Uxbridge
Middlesex UB8 3PH

Fiona Moffatt
Clinical Specialist Physiotherapist
Critical Care Outreach Team
Nottingham University Hospital
Queens Medical Centre Campus
Nottingham NG7 2UH

Stephanie Tempest
Lecturer in Occupational Therapy
School of Health Sciences and
    Social Care
Brunel University
Mary Seacole Building
Uxbridge
Middlesex UB8 3PH

Sandra Naylor
Director of Physiotherapy
School of Health Sciences and
    Social Care
Brunel University
Mary Seacole Building
Uxbridge
Middlesex UB8 3PH

Nicola Plastow
Lecturer in Occupational Therapy
School of Health Sciences and Social
    Care
Brunel University
Mary Seacole Building
Uxbridge
Middlesex UB8 3PH

Chapter 1:

Anita Atwal
Lecturer in Occupational Therapy
School of Health Sciences and
    Social Care
Brunel University
Mary Seacole Building
Uxbridge
Middlesex UB8 3PH

Wolfie Smith
Physical Disability Service
    Manager Camden,
Camden PCT
Peckwater Centre

6 Peckwater Street
London NW5 2TX

Chapter 2:

Mandy Jones & Alison Warland
Lecturers in Physiotherapy
School of Health Sciences and
    Social Care
Brunel University
Mary Seacole Building
Uxbridge
Middlesex UB8 3PH

Chapter 3:

Alison Blank
Lecturer in Occupational Therapy
School of Health Sciences and
    Social Care
Brunel University
Mary Seacole Building
Uxbridge
Middlesex UB8 3PH

Chapter 4:

Thelma Sumsion
Associate Professor for the School
    of Occupational Therapy at
    the University of Western Ontario
Elborn College
University of Western Ontario
London
Ontario, Canada, N6G 1H1

Chapter 5:

Margaret Gallagher
Lecturer in Occupational Therapy
School of Health Sciences and
    Social Care
Brunel University
Mary Seacole Building
Uxbridge
Middlesex UB8 3PH

Elizabeth Cassidy
Lecturer in Physiotherapy
School of Health Sciences and
    Social Care
Brunel University
Mary Seacole Building
Uxbridge
Middlesex UB8 3PH

Chapter 6:

Kee Hean Lim
Lecturer in Occupational Therapy
School of Health Sciences and
    Social Care
Brunel University
Mary Seacole Building
Uxbridge
Middlesex UB8 3PH

Chapter 7:

David Anderson-Ford
Senior Lecturer in Health Studies and
    Health Care Ethics
School of Health Sciences and
    Social Care
Brunel University
Mary Seacole Building
Uxbridge
Middlesex UB8 3PH

Chapter 8:

Anne McIntyre
Lecturer in Occupational Therapy
School of Health Sciences and
    Social Care
Brunel University
Mary Seacole Building
Uxbridge
Middlesex UB8 3PH

Chapter 9:

Sally Spencer
Lecturer in Health Studies

School of Health Sciences and
  Social Care
Brunel University
Mary Seacole Building
Uxbridge
Middlesex UB8 3PH

Chapter 10:

Margaret Gallagher
Lecturer in Occupational Therapy
School of Health Sciences and
  Social Care
Brunel University
Mary Seacole Building
Uxbridge
Middlesex UB8 3PH

Chapter 11:

Mandy Jones
Lecturer in Physiotherapy
School of Health Sciences and
  Social Care

Brunel University
Mary Seacole Building
Uxbridge
Middlesex UB8 3PH

Judith McIntyre
Senior Career Advisor
1st Floor – Bannerman Centre
Brunel University
Mary Seacole Building
Uxbridge
Middlesex UB8 3PH

Chapter 12:

Christine Craik
Director of Occupational Therapy
School of Health Sciences and
  Social Care
Brunel University
Mary Seacole Building
Uxbridge
Middlesex UB8 3PH

Contributors' biographies

David Anderson-Ford

Senior Lecturer at Brunel University, specialising in Healthcare Law and Ethics. He created the first Departmental Research Ethics Committee at Brunel nearly 20 years ago and is Chair of the University Research Ethics Committee. He is a long-standing LREC member, and co-convenor of the UK Universities Research Ethics Working Group. Mr Anderson-Ford is also Chairman Elect of the Association of Research Ethics Committees.

Alison Blank

Lecturer in Occupational Therapy at Brunel University. She has worked in clinical practice for many years, principally in the field of adult mental health. She has been extensively involved in the dissemination of the training manual, Psychosis Revisited. This is a two-day workshop for mental health workers, service users and carers which provides a reflective space for those involved with people who experience psychosis.

Elizabeth Cassidy

Lecturer in Physiotherapy at Brunel University. She has a Masters in Neuro-rehabilitation and extensive clinical experience in the field of adult brain injury rehabilitation. She is specifically interested in the rehabilitation approaches for people with ataxia and working in partnership with patients and carers in education and research.

Christine Craik

Director of Occupational Therapy at Brunel University. Her career has included extensive clinical and management experience in mental health and in occupational therapy education. She is a past Chairman of the

British Association and College of Occupational Therapists. She presents at national and international conferences and publishes her research on mental health, management and occupational therapy education. Her current research includes inpatients' perspectives of occupational engagement in forensic mental health units.

Margaret Gallagher

Lecturer in Occupational Therapy at Brunel University. She has considerable experience of the management of occupational therapy and other professions in the NHS, in acute, community and mental health settings. Her experience in education has encompassed practice education, continuing professional development and quality assurance in education as a reviewer for the Quality Assurance Agency in Higher Education. Her research interests include the involvement of patients and carers in the design and delivery of healthcare programmes, interprofessional learning and clinical supervision in practice. She is a past vice chairman of COT. Her practice experience has been primarily with children with disabilities.

Mandy Jones

Lecturer in physiotherapy, School of Health Sciences and Social Care, Brunel University, London. She has a Doctoral Degree in Physiology from Imperial College of Medicine, Science and Technology, a Masters in Physiology from University College London and a Graduate Diploma in Physiotherapy. Her career has included extensive clinical experience in critical care and respiratory medicine plus physiotherapy education. She published an applied physiology text book aimed at physiotherapists, which is now a core text nationally at undergraduate level. She wrote the curriculum and coordinated the first multiprofessional MSc in adult critical care. Her special interest is the influence of sleep on respiratory physiology, which continues to be her research focus.

Kee Hean Lim

Lecturer in Occupational Therapy at Brunel University. He has extensive experience of working in mental health. He has been involved in several consultations on behalf of the College of Occupational Therapists, within the area of Cultural and Professional practice. He is also a member of the National Steering Group on Delivering Race Equality in Mental Health. His current research interests include cultural sensitivity in practice, sociocultural construction of occupational therapy and occupation, service user inclusion and involvement and the Kawa model. He has presented and delivered papers and workshops within these areas, both at a national and international level.

Anne McIntyre

Lecturer in Occupational Therapy at Brunel University. She is currently undertaking her doctoral research exploring a client-centred falls management programme for older people with dementia. Previous clinical experience was in neurological and older rehabilitation, paediatrics, working in multidisciplinary and inter-agency teams. Scholarly activity includes joint editorship of *Occupational Therapy and Older People* with Anita Atwal, project management and production of guidelines on the WHO's ICF and Health Promotion for the College of Occupational Therapists, article reviewer for the British Journal of Occupational Therapy and a book reviewer for Blackwell Publishing, as well as national and international publications and conference presentations.

Judith McIntyre

Senior careers adviser at Brunel University with 15 years experience. She worked as a careers officer in schools and a further education college for a number of years before moving into higher education. A former nurse, she has spent much of her time at Brunel advising physiotherapy students, visiting physiotherapy recruiters and working with the university's physiotherapy department to develop its careers management modules. She has a Doctorate in Education, an MA in Education and a degree in Sociology. An active member of the Association of Graduate Careers Advisory Services, she is a member of its Education Liaison Task Group.

Sandra Naylor

Senior Lecturer at Brunel University. She is the Director of Physiotherapy Studies in the School of Health Sciences and Social Care. Her main research interests include: physiotherapy education, including newly qualified physiotherapists' expectations and experiences of their first posts; public involvement in healthcare education; and qualitative approaches to research.

Nicola Plastow

Lecturer at Brunel University since September 2005. She graduated from the University of Cape Town, South Africa, in 2000 and moved to the UK working initially as an occupational therapist with older people in a variety of clinical settings in Lancashire, Yorkshire and London. Her area of interest is older people with mental health problems. While in Yorkshire, she completed an MSc in Professional Health Studies at York St. John University and has subsequently published her research on the continuing professional development of occupational therapists working in multidisciplinary teams. Her current doctoral studies focus on the relationship between ageing, food-related occupations and the maintenance of identity.

Shari Rone-Adams

Lecturer in Physiotherapy and Coordinator of Clinical Education at the School of Health Sciences and Social Care, Brunel University, London. She has a Doctoral Degree in Business Administration from Nova Southeastern University, Ft. Lauderdale, FL, and a BS in Physical Therapy from University of Miami, Coral Gables, FL. Dr. Rone-Adams has been involved in clinical education for over 20 years both as a clinical educator and then as clinical coordinator at university level. Her background includes physiotherapy work in the United States in a variety of settings as clinician, manager/administrator and consultant, with a specialisation in geriatrics.

Wolfie Smith

Physical Disability Service Manager at the Camden Physical Disability and Brain Injury Team (an integrated health and social care team), the Camden and Islington Wheelchair Service and the Camden Direct Access Physiotherapy Service. He is a Physiotherapy Clinical Specialist in Neurology and Physical Disability Specialist, and has an interest in older people's rehabilitation and community-based neurological rehabilitation.

Sally Spencer

Lecturer in Health Studies at Brunel University. Responsible for postgraduate teaching focusing on research methods and evidence-based healthcare. She is a member of the Admissions, Marketing and Recruitment Committee and a co-opted member of the Research Ethics Committee. She is the supervisor of two doctoral research students in the field of health services and patient-reported outcomes research. She remains active in research investigating outcomes measurement and clinical trials. She is a research consultant to several pharmaceutical companies, and is currently co-authoring the Cochrane Collaboration systematic review in an aspect of chronic obstructive pulmonary disease.

Thelma Sumsion

Director of the School of Occupational Therapy at the University of Western Ontario in London, Ontario, Canada. She has been working, teaching and researching client-centred practice for over 30 years and has many publications to her credit on this topic. She is the editor of a book titled *Client-Centred Practice in Occupational Therapy: A Guide to Implementation*, that is now in its second edition. She has worked and studied in both Canada and England and has recently been appointed as an adjunct professor at the University of Limerick.

Introduction

Making the transition from student to qualified graduate is a challenging time for any healthcare professional. Most enter their chosen profession with a mixture of both enthusiasm and trepidation; maintaining a duty of care to service users and the responsibility of clinical decision making are some of the criteria embedded in being a healthcare professional. These and many other associated qualities and skills are not necessarily inherent, but learnt through experience and continually refined throughout a career; as such, many graduates start their careers feeling unprepared. We decided to write this book for numerous reasons, but predominantly to give new healthcare professionals insight and guidance, promoting confidence and proficiency in order to deliver high-quality patient care. We are both passionate about our professions and would like future healthcare professionals to continue to develop and extend the scope of both physiotherapy and occupational therapy. We believe this book will help students and clinicians reflect upon and resolve professional issues, by providing them with a practical and strategic approach to their practice, career structure and continued professional development.

Sadly, high-quality patient care is not always maintained. Reports of poor patient care appear in the media on an all too regular basis. Indeed, the recent case of Joan Dorling (Skellingrton, 2008) documents the sequential lack of care she received during a National Health Service hospital admission in the United Kingdom. Her daughter kept a diary, highlighting areas of concern which were fed back to the hospital staff after her death, in an attempt to improve the care received by subsequent patients. The diary documented a series of incidents which on reflection are the antithesis of caring; no attempt to settle Joan in to the ward or make her feel welcome, no access to essential personal belongings such as glasses and a hearing aid, exclusion from discussion, goal setting and management implementation, isolation, unrealistic expectations and poor communication with ward staff.

Dorling's account provides a platform on which to view and reflect on the contributing factors to her mother's unsatisfactory experience of hospitalisation. These include a breakdown in core components integral to healthcare provision: professionalism, client centred-practice, patient dignity, patient autonomy, communication and teamwork, healthcare documentation and, above all, the ability to reflect on and continually develop clinical practice. These areas provide a focus for this book which extends to discuss many of the challenges and complexities associated with multi-professional working in an ever evolving healthcare environment. Professional practice is continually developing in response to health and social care policy, evolving technology and patient requirement. So we asked our colleagues to reflect upon the current and future challenges to clinical practice as a healthcare professional. Naylor and Rhone Adams discuss the meaning of professionalism, whilst Moffatt focuses on professionalism itself. Tempest and Plastow identify the key aspects of challenges to professional practice, namely paid occupation, belonging, competency and skill, all of which are components of professionalism. Finally, Harvey gives a personal account of the pride and satisfaction she associates with being a healthcare professional.

Being professional
Sandra Naylor and Shari Rone-Adams

As a member of a profession there is an assumption that a practitioner will always demonstrate professionalism in all aspects of their lives. However, consensus in defining professionalism is difficult to find (Parker et al, 2006). In the health arena most definitions of professionalism include respect for the patient, altruism, integrity and advocacy (DuToit, 1995; Parker et al, 2006). Hunt et al (1998: 266) describe professionalism as 'the application of a set of principles, attitudes and behaviour standards and patterns to the practice of the discipline'.

All practitioners must have integrity; integrity is a core value of professionalism. Its key elements are adherence to high ethical and professional standards, truthfulness, honesty, and doing what you say you will do (American Physical Therapy Association, 2008). In some instances there may be cases when you are obliged to break confidentiality in order to prevent harm to someone else, i.e. in some cases there may be competing moral principles. Professionals have a duty to promote social responsibility, which means promoting cultural competence as well as maintaining moral, legal and humanistic principles. Hence professionals need to support and promote availability and access to healthcare, and support fairness and non-discrimination in the delivery of care.

The Standards of Conduct applied to Clinical Nursing states that *altruism* is a concern for the welfare and well being of others. Altruistic behaviour by a therapist might include, for example, continuing to work outside contracted hours, or a willingness to access all the extra resources to help patients, students and colleagues. In fact, altruism is based around the principles of professionals working unselfishly, although in practice this can sometimes be difficult.

Compassion and caring are under-utilised words in the therapy professions. Caring is the concern, empathy and consideration for the needs and values of others. Hence in practice this means being client centred as we are empowering clients to the highest levels. On a more practical level this means ensuring that the patient's basic needs are always met and that their dignity is maintained at all times. Compassion is the desire to identify with or sense something of other people's experiences and is regarded as a precursor for caring.

The American Physical Therapy Association (2008: 4) refers to professional duty as 'meeting one's obligations to providence effective physical therapy services to patients/clients to service the profession and to positively influence the health of society'. It involves becoming involved within professional activities, such as attending conferences or organising study days or even reviewing for your professional journal. More over, it requires clinicians to know and understand best evidence, and to ensure that competencies, that are set by the professional and healthcare organisations in which we practise, are met. Competencies define not only what a person must know and do, but also how a person behaves. Competencies typically include a definition and some observable behaviours that, when performed, may indicate acceptable performance. Competencies help align the stakeholders (teachers, students, professionals, patients) with the evidence based principles that guide professional application of speciality standards (Verma et al, 2006).

The meaning of professionalism
Fiona Moffatt

Professionalism is a personal and experiential concept. Influential mentors and role models initially mould our opinions and provide clinicians with a benchmark to aspire to. We can all cite colleagues who have inspired us over our academic and working lives (just as we can recall those whose behaviour has made us question their professionalism).

My personal concept of professionalism is defined by a core set of values, behaviours and standards with which I have chosen to practise my vocation. Integral to these values is the commitment to clinical credibility and competence, moral and ethical integrity, seeking excellence and awareness of reasonable scope of practice. Compassion, mutual trust and respect (for patients and colleagues) and promoting continual personal development via evaluation of practice and demonstration of learning and research are also essential. The authority of a professional body, which guides, directs and regulates me as an individual, but also engenders public esteem and confidence, reinforces this personal infrastructure.

Over the years I have witnessed a climate change in the approach to professionalism. It is widely accepted that modern professionalism is viewed as a partnership, engaging patient, clinician, the healthcare system and interactions therein (Doctors in Society, 2005). The dated model of a hierarchical team with a senior professional that 'knew best' has been replaced with a dynamic approach, which fosters accountability and openness, shares responsibility and acknowledges the necessity of life-long learning. Equally, the public's perception of professionalism has shifted. In this technological and media-orientated era, health professionals often find themselves the subject of a scrutinising spotlight. There has been a great shift in expectations of the public, with an ever-increasing emphasis on consumerism, further fuelled by readily available medical information via the Internet. Professionalism dictates that clinicians respond to this challenge, viewing it as a method of empowering and engaging the public, rather than a threat to their credibility. Similarly, political influences and financial constraints often constitute a challenge to professionalism. Acknowledging that a 'value-for-money' approach to healthcare provision is essential, professionals must be cognisant of the necessity for judicious use of resources whilst ensuring that they take an active role in service organisation and deployment of such valued assets.

Given the background of radical change in healthcare delivery, it is therefore essential that clinicians and teams continue to re-examine and redefine those traits that encapsulate professionalism in the modern NHS.

Professional practice: belonging, paid occupation, competent and skilful
Stephanie Tempest and Nicola Plastow

On contemplating how to approach our task for this introduction, we sought guidance from our trusted friend, The Oxford English Dictionary (OED). It defines professional as:

1. relating or belonging to a profession;
2. engaged in a sport or other activity as a paid occupation;
3. appropriate to a professional person; competent or skilful.

We felt the key ingredients within this definition for us as healthcare professionals were: belonging, paid occupation, competent and skilful. So, we decided to base our personal reflections on these four topics when considering what professional practice means to us.

Belonging

'Belonging' is both extrinsic and intrinsic in nature. On an extrinsic level, we belong to others: to our service users, our student cohorts, our chosen healthcare professions, our multidisciplinary teams and the organisation that employs us. Continuing to 'belong' to those we work with as professionals requires a clear commitment to our professional roles; a willingness to meet the needs and expectations of others by going the extra mile, and adaptability to the changes that inevitably occur at every level of practice. A sense of extrinsic belonging brings responsibility and expectations from others.

On an intrinsic level, we have to identify with and feel at ease within our chosen profession. We need to identify with our 'brand' and take pride in developing our professional role, but not at the expense of others. We need to develop and maintain an intrinsic sense of what we are able to offer and where we link with others. Part of this is having a clear understanding of what makes your profession 'special' and what your professional skills are that no other member of your team can offer. We believe it is essential, for us as individuals and as healthcare professions, to understand who we are, where we have come from, where we want to get to and how we are going to get there. A sense of intrinsic belonging brings responsibility and expectations from within.

Paid occupation

Being a healthcare professional means getting paid for what we do. Payment can take the form of wages, student bursaries or scholarships. What you are paid confers a certain status, and to a certain extent also determines the level of responsibility you are required to carry within an organisation, particularly a large one like the NHS. We must remember that we are paid to produce and deliver the goods, whether this is delivering an assignment on time as a student or providing a reliable and effective service as a practitioner. In this context, we believe professional practice means we must earn our keep.

At the same time our paid occupations are not our only valued occupations. We believe there is a balance to be found. This balance is essential in order to sustain our professional practice over time; maintain our passion and enthusiasm for meeting the needs of our service users, particularly at times of difficulty; and in developing ourselves as people, not just as professionals.

Competent

In order to claim professional practice, we must have the skills and the knowledge to do something successfully. Becoming, being and staying a competent practitioner does not happen by accident or fortune. It is no longer an option to complete undergraduate training as a professional and never again update our practice with new knowledge that has evolved during our careers.

We believe that competence is an evolving concept that must be aimed for at every level within our professional career. We need to recognise our own incompetence in order to work hard to develop skills and knowledge, for example as an undergraduate student or when entering a new area of professional practice. We also need to recognise when we have achieved a high level of competence, for example when seeking promotion.

A competent, professional practitioner is someone who actively seeks to develop their knowledge and skills through a broad range of both formal and informal learning opportunities. The competent professional then reflects on these activities and successfully advances and develops their practice with the new knowledge gained.

Skilful

Every profession has its own set of core skills in which a high level of competence is essential. There are also other skills that all healthcare professionals share. Being a professional practitioner is about having and showing a range of skills. Some skills are basic, such as completing a report on time or following protocols; some are highly skilful and complex, for example utilising reflective and empathetic skills when discussing weekend leave with an anxious relative.

The way forward

If these are the key ingredients for professional practice, there is one question left: how do we achieve this in practice?

Our advice, for all of us, is that professional practice is about keeping an enquiring and open mind, thus minimising the risk of falling into a routine and prescriptive 'one size fits all' approach to study and work. It is through enquiry that we will become and remain professional. Being professional means maintaining a sense of extrinsic and intrinsic belonging; being skilful and having the ability to do something well; being knowledgeable and competent; and deserving the money that is invested in us.

What does being a health professional mean to me?
Alex Harvey

What does being a health professional mean to me? Well, the first word that springs to mind is pride. I was incredibly proud to become a qualified physiotherapist 14 years ago and I still am to this day. I really believe in my profession and the vital part they have to play in the healthcare system.

Why am I proud of my profession? I believe that we operate to incredibly high standards of practice. The profession is now aware of the need for a sound evidence base and is not afraid to adapt so as to meet the changing needs of the healthcare system. We are moving with the times, and in my opinion our knowledge, skills and ability to provide excellent patient care are improving all the time.

What is the best part of being a healthcare professional? For me, there is no greater feeling than leaving work at the end of the day knowing you have made a real difference to a patient's experience. It may be that you have reinflated a patient's lung and therefore prevented them from being intubated on intensive care. Or it may simply be that you have spent an extra 10 minutes with a patient who needed to talk. Whichever it is, the poor salary and unpaid overtime all become worthwhile when a patient thanks you personally for your care and attention.

What are the future challenges for my profession? I believe we must continue to embrace extended scope practice so that we can gain the necessary skills to improve patient care. We are not losing our professional identity, simply evolving to meet the needs of the healthcare system. The drive for high-quality research must continue and this should commence at undergraduate level. Indeed, physiotherapy students must be taught evidence-based practice and be encouraged to challenge clinical practice where appropriate.

What would be my advice to students about to embark on their career in a healthcare profession? I think the most important thing is to always maintain your standards. Follow the example of expert practitioners that have inspired you. By giving 100% you will be able to take great pride in your work and the level of care that you provide. Having said all that, don't take work too seriously. Work really should be fun and having a good giggle with your colleagues is essential to this.

References

American Physical Therapy Asociation (2008) Ethics and Legal Resources. http://www.apta.org/AM/Template.cfm?Section=Ethics_and_Legal_Issues1&Template=/TaggedPage/TaggedPageDisplay.cfm&TPLID=48&ContentID=4116 (Accessed 6th December 2008).

Doctors in Society (2005) Medical professionalism in a CHANGING world. London: Royal College of Physicians.

Du Toit, D. (1995) A sociological analysis of the extent and influence of professional socialization on the development of a nursing identity among nursing students at two universities in Brisbane, Australia. Journal of Advanced Nursing 21(1), 164–171.

Hunt, A., Higgs, J., Adamson, B., Harris, L. (1998) University education and the physiotherapy professional. Physiotherapy 84(6), 264–273.

Parker, K., Moyo, E., Boyd, L., Hewitt, S., Weltz, S., Reynolds, S. (2006) What is professionalism in the applied health sciences? Journal of Allied Health 35(20), 91–102.

Skellington, D. (2008) *Catalogue of Disaster*. The Guardian. Wednesday 28 May http://www.guardian.co.uk/theguardian (Accessed 29th May 2008).

Verma, S., Paterson, M., Medves, J. (2006) Core competencies for healthcare professionals. *Journal of Allied Health* **35**(2), 109–115.

World Health Organization (2001) *International Classification of Functioning, Disability and Health*. Geneva: World Health Organization.

1: Interprofessional teamwork

Anita Atwal and Wolfie Smith

In the allied health professions there is an acknowledgement that the transition from graduate to clinician can be challenging. The transition from student to practitioner requires health professionals to work as an effective team member within complex organisations. Hence clinicians need to posses a wide range of hard and soft skills. Hard skills refer to problem solving, clinical expertise, critical thinking and self-reflection, whilst soft skills refer to skills such as time management, listening, ability to get on with people, empathy and networking skills. The issue is whether interprofessional working is of any benefit to the growth and promotion of the allied health professions? What are the current trials and tribulations of teamwork? How can teams work effectively? This chapter outlines the problems of interprofessional practice in health and social care. It examines the meaning of teamwork, why interprofessional working is important, factors that impact upon teamworking, how to resolve team issues and how to manage conflict or difficult situations in teams. Examples from research based in practice will be used to analyse such problems, how they arose and ways in which they might be addressed.

Membership and composition of teams

Multidisciplinary teams were formulated in order to respond to the changes which were occurring in medicine in the 1950s and 1960s, namely the growth of 'holistic' medicine (Brown, 1982). Teams were perceived to be the most effective means to manage the patient's social, medical, psychological, cognitive, environmental and rehabilitative needs. Teams are considered to have numerous advantages over traditional care. The frequently cited advantages include improved planning, more clinically effective services, a more responsive and patient-focused service, avoidance of duplication and fragmentation and more satisfying roles for healthcare professionals (Royal Pharmaceutical Society of Great Britain and British Medical Association, 2000). In some cases, multidisciplinary teams may not have an outcome that can be measured (Box 1.1).

Most therapists, nurses, doctors and social workers become members of a team by default, i.e. the post which they occupy requires them to work in a multidisciplinary team. Consequently we do not choose who

> **Box 1.1** Multidisciplinary teams need to have clear outcomes
>
> Multidisciplinary team meetings that do not have an outcome that can be meas-
> ured can be viewed as ineffective (Atwal, 2002). This is a view of a staff nurse:
>
> > I have been to others (multidisciplinary team meetings) where nothing has
> > been sorted out and everything still remains the same. . .You know seven
> > months in an acute hospital bed taking up space when nothing happens.

we work with. Moreover, in most instances support workers and users
of services are often excluded from team meetings.

Interestingly, current journal articles regularly fail to include occupational therapy assistants as members of an occupational therapy or
multidisciplinary team; this is a concerning oversight. Effective collaboration between therapists and assistants will be needed to deliver
more effective and responsive care to clients. Therefore it is vital that
therapists develop a good understanding and appreciation of their differing roles and that training is in place to enhance the roles of therapy
assistants.

The exclusion of therapy assistants from team meetings can impact
upon clinical decision making. Our own anecdotal evidence suggests
that despite having valuable information regarding a patient's condition and progress, most healthcare assistants are excluded from team
meetings (Atwal & Jones, 2007). One healthcare assistant told us:

> We are the closest of the staff to the patient so we assess them and we can
> tell, even though we haven't a part to tell anybody else, . . .we know what
> they are capable of doing. They don't ask us, they ask the people who are
> far from them. . . Therefore the assessment is really faulty.

HCAs should be actively encouraged to participate in team meetings,
and supported to do so by their colleagues. This in turn could allow
accurate information to be shared with members of the team, which will
subsequently enhance and improve decision making and, ultimately,
patient care.

Professionals need to consider how the patient voice is heard within
teams. How do we ensure that that the patients' opinions are truly
represented within multidisciplinary teams? How do we feel about or
even manage service users who are assertive and articulate and can
challenge individual members of the teams and the decisions that have
been made about them? Service users are the most important members
of the team, but little research has occurred regarding how they can
be integrated into teams. There is some evidence that involving service users in interprofessional education can enable students to become
more patient centred (Barnes et al, 2006).

Box 1.2 How effective is your team?

How does your profession cultivate teamworking?
What is your experience of teamworking in your organisation?
What kind of team do you work in?
Could it be enhanced?
Do teams work in your setting?

From our own experience, one of the most essential aspects to ensure good partnership working is to develop good listening and communication skills. It is essential that professionals spend time listening to users and can evidence decisions that have been made. Some users are taking the initiative and the time to understand specific health conditions. In the past the emphasis has always been on the healthcare professional imparting information to the service user in conversation and with leaflets. Now the service user will already be well informed with information they have researched and downloaded from the Internet. It is important that healthcare professionals are not threatened by the fact the patient may know extensive detail about their condition. What it does mean is that professionals must be able to effectively evidence their interventions with users (see Chapter 9). It is also important to be aware that service users may think they have insight into their condition, which may actually be misplaced. It can require skill to undertake a conversation explaining that the facts the service user has extracted from Wikipedia are not necessarily comparable to the randomised controlled trial that advocates a specific direction for treatment (Rampil, 1998). Supporting the service user to understand the need to separate the 'wheat' from the 'chaff' on the Internet can be an important part of developing a relationship which enables the user to participate in the service offered.

In clinical practice, we have observed and participated in three different models of teamworking. The first model (which appears to be the norm within acute care settings) is when the patient is absent from all team meetings. The second model is when the consultant performs a bedside ward round and the patient is asked to comment on 'how they are feeling'. Our experience of this model usually results in the patient agreeing to everything the doctor says. The third model, which can occur in psychiatry, is when the patient is asked to attend the team meeting. In this instance, the experience can be daunting for the service user. The question is, if the patient is not a member of the team can you really say that you have adopted a person-centred approach? We would suggest that therapists and other professionals need to consider the use of experts in practice that could act as advocates for patients. Please answer the questions in Box 1.2 about the team you work in or have worked in.

Preparation for teamwork

In order for a team to work effectively, its members must be 'competent to collaborate' (Barr, 1998:183). Barr (1998) has identified competencies which are thought to be necessary for effective interprofessional working:

- contribute to the development and knowledge of others;
- enable practitioners and agencies to work collaboratively;
- develop, sustain and evaluate collaborative approaches;
- contribute to joint planning, implementation, monitoring and review;
- coordinate an interdisciplinary team;
- provide assessment of needs so that others can take action;
- evaluate the outcome of another practitioner's assessment.

The need for pre-qualifying education to prepare students to work as part of a team has been clearly articulated (Miller et al, 1999; Barr, 2000). However, opportunities for interprofessional education are far scarcer in relation to pre-qualifying educational programmes than in post-qualification (Koppel et al, 2001). One of the major difficulties in considering interprofessional education is the lack of clarity in the use of terminology (Cooper et al, 2001). A systematic review on interdisciplinary education of undergraduate healthcare professional students found that student healthcare professionals benefited from interdisciplinary education with outcome effects relating mainly to changes in knowledge, skills, attitudes and beliefs. However, effects upon professional practice were not apparent (Cooper et al, 2001). At present, the research available into the effectiveness of interprofessional education is contradictory and there is little evidence to demonstrate its effectiveness (Zwarenstein et al, 1999, 2001). In the literature some authors argue that interprofessional education enhances motivation to collaborate (Barr 1998; Parsell et al 1998), contributes to the development of effective collaborative teamwork (Freeth & Reeves 2000) and overcomes prejudice and negative stereotypes (Carpenter 1995). On the other hand, it has been suggested that interprofessional education reinforces negative attitudes and stereotypes and that it may encourage role confusion and loss of professional expertise (Tope, 1996; Leaviss, 2000). In addition, educators themselves can reinforce negative stereotypes and prejudices which can hinder interprofessional learning (Barr, 2000). Besides, opinion varies concerning the timing of interprofessional education. It has been suggested that it should take place at pre-registration level to mitigate the risk of developing negative attitudes and to prepare future healthcare professionals to work effectively as team members (Miller et al, 1999; Freeth & Reeves, 2000).

The terminology associated with 'shared learning', such as 'interprofessional', 'collaborative' and 'multiprofessional', is often used interchangeably. The authors make a clear distinction between multiprofessional

Box 1.3 Do you have the skills needed to be an effective team player?

Are you competent to collaborate?
What additional skills/training do you need to be a competent team player?
How will you acquire such skills?

education as 'simply learning together' and interprofessional education as 'learning together to promote collaborative practice', and relate this closely to the distinction made between multidisciplinary and interprofessional practice. Consequently newly qualified practitioners can be unprepared for teamwork in the real world. Please answer the questions in Box 1.3 about your own collaborative skills.

Perceptions of teamwork

Within the health and social services the term multidisciplinary is used to denote almost any form of cooperation between professionals and agencies. Hence multidisciplinary teamwork may be regarded as everyone performing his or her own thing with little or no awareness of other disciplines' work. This confusion regarding what is meant by teamworking has arisen from the miscellaneous terms which have been used to represent the multidisciplinary team concept (Coleman, 1982; Mariano, 1989). The reason for this is that the resemblance of a 'team' masks the range and complexity possible in interdisciplinary interaction and cooperation (Kane, 1983; Gregson et al, 1991). Occupational therapists' and physiotherapists' perceptions of teams have not been researched in great detail. One study (Atwal & Caldwell, 2006) found that there was remarkable scepticism surrounding the concept of the multidisciplinary team. Nurses described the multidisciplinary team as a 'complete myth', 'idealistic' and 'shambolic'.

There have been many attempts to define collaboration, which, once again like the term multidisciplinary, can be defined according to those implementing the concept; this has resulted in a superficial definition (Kraus, 1980). Webb (1986:155) refers to collaboration as:

> The pursuit of a coordinated course of actions usually through face to face interaction by means of achieving consensus about a field of interests and goals which are to be furthered by mutually acceptable means.

Armitage (1983) has introduced taxonomy of collaboration within five stages which is helpful since it measures and defines collaboration. The first stage is isolation, where members never meet, talk or write to one another. The second stage is where members communicate with each

Box 1.4 Can integrated care pathways enhance teamworking?

This study evaluated multidisciplinary integrated care pathways to improve inter-professional collaboration (Atwal & Caldwell, 2002). It was part of a larger action research study to analyse and improve multidisciplinary teamwork and discharge planning. Integrated care pathways are interdisciplinary plans of the outline optimal sequencing and timing of interventions for patients with a particular diagnosis, procedure or symptom (Ignatavicius & Hausman, 1995). They were believed to develop multidisciplinary teamworking (de Luc, 2000). This research study found that integrated care pathways did not enhance interprofessional collaboration and that professionals did not regard recording team goals as a priority. Moreover the study highlighted the need for effective documentation; if the notes were not completed, communication was fragmented. However the implementation of integrated care pathways did improve the quality of the management of the patient and reduced length of stay.

other but do not interact meaningfully. The third stage is concerned with communication which includes the exchange of information. The fourth stage is partial collaboration where members who act on that information sympathetically participate in patterns of joint working and subscribe to the same general objectives as others on a one-to-one basis in the same organisation. The fifth stage is full collaboration which occurs in an organisation where the work of all members is fully integrated.

Within your own team it is essential to explore the many definitions in order to ascertain whether these terms are distinguishable or one and the same. Moreover it is essential to ascertain whether all team members perceive teamwork in the same way. However, teamworking is a sensitive area and other members of the team may not wish to acknowledge that there is an underlying problem. Hence in our experience, the first hurdle of any change or exploration work is to discuss informally with key stakeholders your feeling and perceptions. It has also been suggested that team members must be involved in developing criteria to assess the competence of the various professional members and the effectiveness of each contribution (Kane, 1983). Box 1.4 outlines a study which evaluated the impact of integrated care pathways on interprofessional collaboration.

Integrative and transdisciplinary teams

The term multidisciplinary has further evolved into the 'integrative' and the 'transdisciplinary' approach which is the most advanced and sophisticated form of teamwork (Woodruf & McGoniegel, 1988; Orelove & Sobsey, 1991). The unique features of an integrative team are that the whole team makes decisions together, so that professionalism is levelled, and that there is shifting leadership focus according to the needs of a particular patient (United Cerebral Palsy, 1976). The concept central to both these models is that of role blurring and role release (Lyon & Lyon, 1980). Thus each individual member of the team is involved in role extension that is improving the clinical knowledge skills in one discipline. Each member of the team is involved in role enrichment, which entails learning about other roles and disciplines, whilst role exchange is learning and beginning to implement techniques from other disciplines. Once these skills are acquired they are then released, which involves putting newly acquired techniques into practice with consultation from team members. In addition other members of the team offer role support in order to allow the role expansion to be successful.

The key aspects of interdisciplinary, integrative and transdisciplinary models is the foundation of 'patient-focused care'. Heyman and Culling (1994:3) point out that there is no single definition for patient-focused care or patient-centred care:

> ...Their thrust is to shorten or eliminate process steps and ease administration and co-ordination burden through limiting the number of staff involved with each patient.

It calls for traditional professional skill boundaries to be re-appraised, the roles of staff to be redesigned, and cross-skilling and multi-skilling, which allow members of care teams to deliver a wide range of services according to the patient's needs and requirements (Lehmann-Spitzer & Yahn, 1992).

Components of unsuccessful teams

The NHS Plan (Department of Health, 2000) has encouraged professionals to consider implementing role integration in healthcare teams. This involves professionals developing new roles as well as sharing skills with members of the multidisciplinary team. There is considerable evidence that unsuccessful teams occur because they are composed of members with undefined roles (Belbin, 1981). Hence it has been suggested that successful teams consist of individuals who not only know their professional roles but also know their own individual style of working in a team. For example you may be a person who enjoys solving difficult problems but is a poor communicator or a person who is well organised and makes ideas happen in practice. On the other hand you may be someone who has lots of energy but can be insensitive to the needs of others. Hence within any team there needs to be an awareness of individual personalities and an understanding of the roles people within the team are fulfilling. This may lead to the identification that a particular characteristic is missing from the team, which if, undertaken and fulfilled, may lead to rapid acceptance into the team. However, beware of trying to fulfil a role that is already successfully filled within that team. In particular, avoid trying to fulfil a role for which several people are already competing. It is unlikely this will be accepted by the team, but instead will contribute to irresolvable conflict (see http://www.belbin.com/downloads/Belbin_Team_Role_Summary_ Descriptions.pdf).

Thus ambiguity and overlap within the health profession can be one of the difficulties in developing teamwork (Cass, 1978). One of the key problems associated with interprofessional conflict is role perception. Forsyth (1990:495) defines a role as 'a behaviour characteristic of persons in a context; the part played by a member of a group'. However Burr (1975:833) is of the opinion that a rigid role may be used by insecure member of the team 'as a basis for demarcation disputes'. In order for professionals to gain an understanding of the roles of other professionals it is essential that they are able to clearly state their role within the healthcare team. Pritchard (1981) notes that the lack of clarity of roles within a multidisciplinary team leads to the development of stereotypical attitudes. Stereotyping is defined by William and William (1982:17) as an 'attempt by an individual to understand his or her social environment'. One study (Dalley & Sim, 2001) found that nurses perceived that physiotherapists did not understand the external pressures that they operated within and that there was a lack of awareness of nurses' professional autonomy and decision making in rehabilitation. Box 1.5 outlines a study by Pietroni (1991) which examined stereotypes in medical, nursing and social work students.

Box 1.5 Archetypes and stereotypes

Pietroni (1991) undertook a study of medical students, nursing and social work students to examine stereotypes and archetypes, and found unexpressed archetypes and stereotypes. At Brunel university we undertake a similar exercise based on the work of Pietroni, but ask students to complete a questionnaire before and after an interprofessional model.
We ask students to write:

What car do you think occupational therapists, physiotherapists, social workers, nurses and doctors drive?
What sort of clothes do they wear?
What newspaper do they read?
What do they do?
What do they do in their spare time?
Can you describe their personalities?
How would you describe occupational therapists, physiotherapists, social workers, nurses and doctors?
How would you describe their team-playing skills?
Do you perceive occupational therapists, physiotherapists, social workers, nurses and doctors as being interested in interprofessional working?

Temporal–spatial and social factors

Developing and sustaining interprofessional relationships are further complicated by temporal–spatial challenges. Due to the nature of professional practice, health and social care practitioners often work in different clinics, wards or organisations at different times of the day (and night). As effective interprofessional collaboration is dependent on open channels of communication, the incompatible working hours of the different professions may result in much of their work being hidden from the eyes of others. Consequently, it is essential that team members spend time with one another to understand each other's roles and their preferred methods of working. In health and social care this can be difficult since professionals rotate at different times and spend limited periods within each speciality (Atwal & Jones, 2007). Consequently it is essential that senior members of a team invest time enabling professionals to meet different team members. Moreover senior members must lead by example and ensure that they promote the value and importance of the team and do not allow so-called 'more important tasks' to come first.

Weak interaction in teams

Multidisciplinary teams are settings in which assumptions are constantly challenged and where team members can share skills and knowledge (Central Council for the Education and Training of Social Workers, 1989). Mackay (1997:176) found that nurses were often reluctant to voice their opinions even if it was a 'matter of life and death'.

The type and amount of interaction in team meetings can be used as an indication of teamwork. Power and status differentials between the different professionals have been explored and indicated the limited involvement of therapists, social worker/care managers and nurses in multidisciplinary team decision making. Wise et al (1974) concluded that high-status members tended to speak first and most convincingly on all issues. A remarkable finding by Fewttrell and Toms (1985) was that in traditional psychiatric ward rounds medical staff talked considerably more than all the other participants put together. Stein (1967) explored the interaction between doctors and nurses and introduced the concept of the doctor–nurse game. He describes how nurses learn to show initiative and offer significant advice while appearing to defer passively to the doctors' authority. Nurses use subtle non-verbal and cryptic cues which, in retrospect, appear to have been initiated by the doctor. The game ensures that open disagreement is avoided at all costs and has advantages for both parties. The doctors gain from the nurses' knowledge and experience, whilst the nurses gain increased satisfaction from his or her more demanding role. One study (Atwal & Caldwell, 2002) explored the interaction patterns of multidisciplinary teams in orthopaedics, elder

> **Box 1.6** Case study: communication in a team
>
> Rory is a newly qualified occupational therapist working on the medical wards. It is Friday and he has had Norman, aged 67, down to the OT kitchen to demonstrate his ability to make a cup of tea, following a long period of bed rest due to a serious deterioration to his health that was eventually diagnosed as prostate cancer. Whilst working together Norman complains to Rory that he has not been able to go to the toilet all day; he feels he has a full bladder but he just can't go. Rory knows that urine retention is a sign of spinal cord compression and is concerned. He tries to raise the issue with the house officer, Cas. Unfortunately the two of them have never got along, Rory is quite shy and Cas has interpreted his aloofness as incompetence. Rory is unable to convince Cas that there is any cause for concern. When Rory returns to work on Monday, he learns that Norman is permanently paralysed. He had a secondary tumour in his spinal cord. Rory is mortified that his inability to communicate the situation effectively to Cas could have contributed to this situation.
>
> How can the situation be resolved?
>
> On his next rotation Rory is working on the elderly rehabilitation wards. Cas is now the senior house officer for these wards. Rory is determined to ensure that no one else comes to harm because of his relationship with Cas. He discusses his problems with his line manager who suggests seeing Cas as a human being first and a doctor second. Rory puts a lot of effort into talking to Cas about things that are unrelated with work. He learns that her grandmother is unwell and always remembers to ask her how she is when they meet. The relationship between them improves.

care and medicine, found that the team was task orientated and suggests that doctors and, in particular, consultants had a more dominant role in teams. Within the nursing team, especially, it was apparent that there was unequal participation between different nurses. However amongst social workers, therapists and nurses similar rates of participation occurred in the different teams. The differing types and amounts of interaction that occurred in all four teams may suggest that the teams were not working effectively. Professionals may lack confidence to voice opinions and ask for information in team meetings. Hence in practice this means that professionals are not respecting their own individual autonomy or being an effective advocate for the client.

Box 1.6 outlines a case study about Rory, a newly qualified occupational therapist. In this instance communication differences are caused by misunderstandings between two members of the team which impacts upon how a patient is managed by a junior doctor in the team. What would you have done in this instance? What will their relationship be like if they work together in another team?

Communication within physiotherapy and occupational therapy teams

Most newly qualified therapists have a senior member of a team (either a physiotherapist or occupational therapist) as their mentor or line manager.

Box 1.7 Case study: policies, procedures and teamwork

A therapy manager, who likes to run a tight ship, runs a therapy team in the community. He has policies and procedures for everything and expects the therapists within the team to apply them vigorously. Lola has just joined the team as a newly qualified member of staff. She is eager to please but has found it difficult to integrate herself within the team as she finds her peers to be very cliquey. In order to impress and get integrated with her peers she has been applying the policies and procedures to the letter.

Lola has been allocated a 20-year-old wheelchair user, William, who has just started work and needs some assistance with reorganising his exercise routine to fit in with his full-time job. William has requested that he have an appointment outside of normal working hours as he contends that he is not ill and therefore cannot ask for time off work. The therapy department policy states that all home visits must be completed before 16:00 to ensure people get their notes written on the day of the visit and for staff safety. Lola has read the policy and therefore refuses to grant this request. William is forced to ask his employers for time off. They refuse as he has only just started working with them and it confirms all their fears about employing a wheelchair user; they see this as the thin end of the wedge. William is therefore denied his right to treatment due to the inflexibility of the organisation. William makes a complaint about Lola's attitude.

Indeed some therapy teams have removed traditional boundaries and introduced cross-therapy management where physiotherapists are line managed by occupational therapists and vice versa. However, there are instances when policies and procedures can impact upon how teams work and more importantly on how members of teams interact with users of services. For example, the management style of the therapy manager may be strangling flexible working and, more importantly, failing to create a sense of autonomy to the therapists working in the department. The effect means that the principles of client-centred working cannot be implemented. How does one challenge the style of the therapy manager? Box 1.7 outlines a case study about a therapy manager who believes strongly in policies and procedures.

In each team it is essential to establish how you communicate with colleagues within your own professional team. When do team members meet? Are these meeting effective? Can you talk openly and honestly in these meetings without fear of retribution? What do they achieve? How are issues within teams dealt with? When do team members actually get to talk to each other? This means not just about work issues but issues that impact upon work, for example family issues? Do you have a good mentor and access to good clinical supervision?

In the Box 1.8, a grade 5 physiotherapist, Ethan, is unclear about who he communicates with in the team to assist him with the management and treatment of complex patients. Moreover he is being pressurised by other members of the team who have certain expectations regarding

Box 1.8 Case study: caseload management

Ethan has been qualified for nearly a year. He works in a small community hospital that has a two-bedded ITU attached to the surgical ward. He is nearly at the end of his medical rotation that includes covering the ITU beds. Normally he is working with either the medical physiotherapy team leader or the band 6 physiotherapist. However, today the team leader is on a course and the band 6 physiotherapist is absent. Therefore, Ethan is alone with the nurses in ITU. Both cases are complex and beyond Ethan's limited experience. One has a fistula between the oesophagus and trachea and has several pints of Guinness in his lungs. A chest drain is *in situ* and the nurses are asking for Ethan to do something to facilitate expectoration. The other case is a patient with Legionnaire's disease, who is expectorating large blood clots; once again the nurses are expecting Ethan to intervene.

Ethan is very worried, as he does not know who to prioritise or how to treat them. He does not know how to contact the team leader or whether he is even allowed to. He rings the physiotherapy department to explain his plight. He speaks to one of his peers in outpatients who immediately reports the problem to her line manager. Phone calls are made to the medical physiotherapy team leader on her course for advice and to ITU to explain the situation. All the senior In-patient therapists are bleeped and it is determined which of them has the time and the experience to be able to deal with ITU. Another senior is asked to provide support for Ethan for the rest of the day. Work is shared to ensure that it is completed. The extra work means they all finish late at which point it is suggested that a trip to the pub is called for.

his role and competencies. In this instance it is a junior colleague who ensures that members of his team are aware of his difficulties and senior members of the team are supportive. In the first instance, Ethan should have known which senior member he could have contacted for clinical advice and supervision.

It is essential not to forget that therapy assistants play a significant role supporting the work of occupational therapists and physiotherapists. It is our opinion that therapy assistants and healthcare assistants also require effective communication skills (both written and verbal) to work effectively in health and social care. Hence, therapists will also need to consider how they will communicate and interact with these staff while continuing to collaborate with their professional colleagues from medicine, nursing, social work and physiotherapy. Within nursing Spilsbury and Meyer (2004) acknowledged work-related tensions which existed between healthcare assistants and registered nurses, and recognised the potentially negative effects this had on teamworking and subsequent patient care. These authors suggested that a power struggle arose between the two groups as a result of some traditionally viewed 'nursing roles' now being undertaken by healthcare assistants. They state the importance of recognising that potential conflict may occur during the negotiations of roles and duties and advocate that mangers take these issues into consideration when formalising service delivery (Spilsbury & Meyer, 2004).

Conflict

Most professionals do not like conflict, however conflict is a natural part of interprofessional working; within the literature conflict is often regarded as an indicator that teamwork is absent. The Central Council for the Education of Training of Social Workers (1989:9) is unique in that it emphasises the positive aspects of conflict: 'multi-disciplinary teamwork is a two-edged sword'. The tensions and conflicts within it are also its creative force. Janis (1972) identified a 'disease' which infects cohesive groups which he termed groupthink. During groupthink, the members do not voice alternative opinions, therefore the group often makes mistakes which could have been avoided. It is defined by Janis (1982:9) as:

> A mode of thinking that people engage in when they are deeply involved in a cohesive in-group, when the members' striving for unanimity over-rides their motivation to realistically appraise alternative courses of actions.

The causes of groupthink have been identified as cohesiveness, isolation, leadership and decisional stress (Janis, 1972; Janis & Mann, 1977). Very often teams do not have agreed procedures for resolving conflict. Spiegel and Spiegel (1984) found that multidisciplinary meetings resolved such difficulties by each team member recording and submitting therapy plans prior to the multidisciplinary meeting. These and the actual plans made at the meeting were recorded and the data showed that 46% of physicians changed their plans after the meetings.

In practice it is important to understand what motivates each team member. Discussions can be undertaken using words and expressions, which will stimulate them. For example, if you know the consultant is worried about length of stay on his/her ward then you can explain how your way of doing things would have an impact on length of stay in the long term. Even if they do not agree with individuals on the team, make sure you are attentive to listening to their point of view. If you do this well they will do the same for you and they might just hear you say something that causes them to change their mind. Do not allow their disagreement to bring conflict into the relationship you are trying to nurture (Booij, 2007). You might not be achieving much in the short term but in the longer term your perseverance may change things.

Status and power

As a professional, you can be a member of more than one team, where conflicting loyalties may occur. The report *Social Workers: their Role and Tasks* (National Institute of Social Work, 1982:125) warns that 'goodwill is not enough to guarantee adequate collaboration'. It is essential that desired outcomes are reported and agreed as professionals or organisations

Box 1.9 Case study: voicing opinions in a team

Cas's consultant has an old fashioned attitude to his work and believes that therapy has very little to do with people getting better or getting home. Rory has a patient who the consultant was asked to see in A&E. Doris was complaining that her legs were getting weak. Dr Elton told her it was old age and sent her home. She represented at A&E following a fall and was admitted. Dr Elton is annoyed that she was admitted and is determined to send her home as soon as possible as she did not sustain an injury.

Rory is undertaking washing practice with her to assess her ability to manage at home. He asks her to transfer from the porter's chair to the perching stool. Doris tries but her legs give way and Rory is forced to manhandle her back into the porter's chair. As he grabs her trunk she screams very loudly. Once she is safely back in the porter's chair Rory checks whether she was screaming in fear. Doris denies this and says she was in excruciating pain from within her back. She gets a similar pain when she tries to stand but not as bad. Once Doris is back on the ward Rory bleeps Cas and discusses the case with her. He is able to explain how he does not feel that this is ordinary back pain. Cas is much more open to listen to his concerns. She agrees to send Doris for an MRI and to explain to Dr Elton why she supports his concerns regarding Doris. When the results come back they are informed that Doris has a spinal abscess and later it transpires that it is tubercular in origin. Dr Elton thanks Rory for saving his reputation.

may be reluctant to invest scarce resources and energy into developing and maintaining relationships with other organisations, when the potential returns on their investment are unclear or intangible.

When comparing the status of professions it is important to take gender into account. It has been suggested that the high presence of women has actually contributed to their lower autonomy and professional status. Davies (1990) found that the average female physiotherapist is less likely then her male colleague to see herself as an independent practitioner. Mackay (1997) found that male nurses are more likely to question a male doctor than a female doctor.

In the example in Box 1.9, because of Rory's improved interprofessional relationship with Cas, he is able to convince her that further tests are needed. Moreover, Rory has been able to reflect upon his previous experiences and has been able to challenge the professional opinion and attitude of a consultant. Indeed, implementing the realities of client-centred practice in the real world takes courage. However because Rory has voiced his concerns, the client's needs are met and a positive result is obtained.

The leader of the multidisciplinary team is usually a member of the medical profession. Kane (1983) analysed 229 teams and found that a typical team consisted of a group with six to ten members led either by a psychiatrist or a physician. The medical profession, in particular hospital consultants, meet many of the characteristics associated with a leader.

Stogdill (1974), after reviewing 106 studies, found that leaders in relation to other members were higher in achievement, orientation, adaptability, ascendancy, energy levels, responsibility taking, self-confidence and sociability. It was the National Institute of Social Workers (1982) which reported that difficulties in collaboration occurred because of the common assumption that the doctor must always be a leader of any team. A national survey was conducted to compare the structure, purpose and restraints of multidisciplinary teamwork across the UK. The data from the research found that most meetings were still led by a consultant in elder care, orthopaedics and acute medicine (Atwal, 2001).

Conclusion

This chapter has highlighted the complex skills that professionals need to function as competent team members. It is not easy to work in a team, since often team members are different in style, attitude, commitment and work ethic. It is essential that family members are viewed as part of the team and need to be regularly updated and involved in the decision-making process. In order to work effectively it is suggested that you should have the following guidelines (Bachi, 2008):

▩ Do not get into a blaming cycle as teams can blame individuals in a team when things go wrong, for example when a discharge is delayed.
▩ Focus on the present and future.
▩ Hold regular team meetings so that you can reflect on the team's successes and failures to help the team determine where they need to go to improve.
▩ Do not get involved in character assassinations of fellow team members. Talking about team members in private with another team member usually involves the blaming process.
▩ Take responsibility for your individual professional contribution to the team and your own behaviour but not the contribution or roles of your team mates.

From a management perspective the common problem for a newly qualified healthcare professional entering employment in the NHS or Social Services is understanding where they 'fit' in the hierarchy. Even for the most confident newly qualified healthcare professional the organisation and hierarchy can be initially confusing. Managers advocate that new healthcare professionals should aim to 'join in' and express their ideas, as they often have a new and objective view of the service, which is valuable for service development. Managers place importance on any individual's contribution to the team irrespective of their level of experience or duration of service; it is the quality of the ideas and the enthusiasm to put them into practice, which count.

> **Box 1.10** Check list (adapted from the National School Board Association, 2007)
>
> ■ Purpose – does your team share a sense of pride in why the team exists and is this essential in accomplishing its mission and goals?
> ■ Priorities – do your team members know what needs to be done, in what order and by whom to achieve team goals?
> ■ Roles – do team members know their role in achieving tasks and are they able to identify when a more skilful member should be allocated the task?
> ■ Decisions – are authority and decision-making lines clearly understood?
> ■ Conflict – is this dealt with openly and considered important to decision making and personal growth?
> ■ Personal traits – do members feel their unique personalities are appreciated and well utilised?
> ■ Norms – have the group norms for working together been agreed and set and are they regarded as standards for everyone in the team?
> ■ Effectiveness – do team members find team meetings efficient and productive and look forward to the time together?
> ■ Success – do team members clearly know when the team has met with success and share in this equally and proudly?
> ■ Training – are opportunities for feedback and updating skills provided and taken advantage of by team members?

Professionals need to be confident in their own role, be able to clearly articulate their role, be able to exchange and receive information and to be able to use their skills to deal with conflicts and tensions within teams. More importantly this chapter has emphasised the need to consider the role of the patient within the team and to consider ways of ensuring that the patient's voice is heard in the team.

Complete the exercise in Box 1.10 to rate your team against the characteristics needed for a well functioning team.

References

Armitage, S.K. (1983) Joint working in primary health care. *Nursing Times Occassional Paper* **79**(28), 75–78.

Atwal, A. (2001) Structure, aim and constraints of inter-professional working. *British Journal of Therapy and Rehabilitation* **8**(10), 366–370.

Atwal, A. (2002) A world apart: how occupational therapists, nurses and care managers perceive each other in acute health care. *British Journal of Occupational Therapy* **65**(10), 446–452.

Atwal, A., Caldwell, K. (2002) Do multidisciplinary integrated care pathways improve interprofessional collaboration? *Scandinavian Journal of Caring Sciences* **16**(4), 360–367.

Atwal, A., Caldwell, K. (2006) Nurses' perceptions of multidisciplinary team work in acute healthcare. *International Journal of Nursing Practice* **12**(6), 359–365.

Atwal, A., Jones, M. (2007) The importance of the multidisciplinary team. *British Journal of Health Care Assistants* **1**(9), 425–430.

Bachi, R. (2008) *How To Be A Better Team Contributor.* http://work911.com/articles/teamcont.htm (Accessed 2nd June 2008).

Barnes, D., Carpenter, J., Dickinson, C. (2006) The outcomes of partnerships with mental health service users in interprofessional education: a case study. *Health and Social Care in the Community* **14**(5), 426–435

Barr, H. (1998) Competent to collaborate: towards a competency-based model for interprofessional education. *Journal of Interprofessional Care* **12**(2), 181–188.

Barr, H. (2000) *Interprofessional Education*: 1997–2000. London: The UK Centre for the Advancement of Interprofessional Education.

Belbin, M. (1981) *Management Teams, Why They Succeed or Fail.* Oxford: Butterworth and Heinemann.

Booij, L. (2007) Conflicts in operating theatres. *Current Opinion in Anaesthesiology* **20**(2), 152–156

Brown, T. (1982) An historical view of health care teams. In: G.J. Agich (ed) *Responsibility in Health Care.* Boston: Reidel.

Burr, M. (1975) Multidisciplinary health teams. *The Medical Journal of Australia* **2**(29), 833–834.

Carpenter, J. (1995) Doctors and nurses: stereotypes and stereotype change in interprofessional education. *Journal of Interprofessional Care* **9**(2), 151–161.

Cass, S. (1978) The effects of the referral process on hospital patients. *Journal of Advanced Nursing* **3**(6), 563–569.

Central Council for the Education and Training of Social Workers (1989) *Multidisciplinary Teamwork Models of Good Practice.* London: CCETSW.

Coleman, P. (1982) Collaboration between services for the elderly mentally infirm. In: C. Ball, P. Coleman, J. Wright (eds) *The Delivery of Services Main Report* Vol.1. University of Southampton, Southampton: Department of Social Work.

Cooper, H., Carlisle, C., Gibbs, T., Watkins, C. (2001) Developing an evidence base for interdisciplinary learning: a systematic review. *Journal of Advanced Nursing* **35**(2), 228–237.

Dalley, J., Sim, J. (2001) Nurses' perceptions of physiotherapists as rehabilitation team members. *Clinical Rehabilitation* **5**(4), 380–389.

de Luc, K. (2000) Care pathways: an evaluation of their effectiveness. *Journal of Advanced Nursing* **32**(2), 485–496.

Department of Health (2000) *The NHS Plan: A Plan for Investment, A Plan for Reform.* London: HMSO.

Davies, J. (1990) Physiotherapy: where are the men? *Physiotherapy* **76**(3), 132–134.

Fewtrell, W.D., Toms, D.A. (1985) Pattern of discussion in traditional and novel ward round procedures. *British Journal of Medical Psychology* **58**(1), 57–62.

Forsyth, D.R. (1990) *Group Dynamics*, 2nd edn. California: Brook/Cole Publishing Company.

Freeth, D., Reeves, S. (2000) Learning to collaborate. *Nursing Times* **96**(13), 40–41.

Gregson, B., Cartidge, A., Bond, J. (1991) *Interprofessional Collaboration in Primary Health Care Organisations*. Occasional Paper 52. London: The Royal College of General Practitioners.

Heymann, T.D., Culling, W. (1994) *The Patient Focused Approach: A Better Way to Run A Hospital?* Kingston Hospital NHS Trust.

Ignatavicius, D.G., Hausman, K.A. (1995) *Clinical Pathways for Collaborative Practice 1*. Philadelphia: W.B. Saunders Company.

Janis, I.L. (1972) *Victims of Groupthink*. Boston: Houghton-Mifflin.

Janis, I.L. (1982) *Victims of Groupthink*, 2nd edn. Boston: Houghton-Mifflin.

Janis, I.L., Mann, L. (1977) *Decision Making. A Psychological Analysis of Conflict, Choice and Commitment*. New York: Free Press.

Kane, A. (1983) *Interprofessional Teamwork*. New York: Syracuse University.

Koppel, I., Barr, H., Reeves, S., Freeth, D., Hammick, M. (2001) Establishing a systematic approach to evaluating the effectiveness of interprofessional education. *Interdisciplinary Care* **3**(1), 41–49.

Kraus, W.A. (1980) *Collaboration in Organizations Alternative to Hierarchy*. New York: Human Science Press.

Lehmann-Spitzer, R., Yahn, K.J. (1992) Patient needs drive an integrated approach to care. *Nursing Management* **23**(8), 30–31.

Leaviss, J. (2000) Exploring the perceived effect of an undergraduate multiprofessional educational intervention, *Medical Education* **34**(6), 183–186.

Lyon, S., Lyon, G. (1980) Team functioning and staff development. A role release approach to providing integrated educational services for severely handicapped students. *Journal of the Association For The Severely Handicapped* **5**(3), 250–263.

Mackay, L. (1997) *Conflict in care medicine and nursing*. London: Chapman and Hall.

Mariano, C. (1989) The case for interdisciplinary collaboration. *Nursing Outlook* **37**(6), 285–288.

Miller, C., Ross, N., Freeman, M. (1999) *Shared Learning and Clinical Teamwork: New Directions in Education for Multiprofessional Practice*. London: EMB.

National Institute of Social Work (1982) *Social Workers: their Role Social Work and Tasks*. London: Bedford Square Press.

Orelove, F.P., Sobsey, D. (1991) *Educating Children With Multiple Disabilities: A Transdisciplinary Approach*. Baltimore: Paul. H. Brookes.

Parsell, G., Spalding, R., Bligh, J. (1998) Shared goals, shared learning: evaluation of a multiprofessional course for undergraduate students. *Medical Education* **32**(3), 304–311.

Pietroni, P.C. (1991) Stereotypes or archetypes? A study of perceptions amongst health care students. *Journal of Social Work Practice* **5**(1), 61–69.

Pritchard, P. (1981) *Manual of Primary Health Care*. Oxford: Oxford University Press.

Rampil, I. (1998) Medical Information on the Internet. *American Society of Anaesthesiologists Inc* **89**(5), 1233–1245.

Royal Pharmaceutical Society of Great Britain and the British Medical Association (2000) *Teamworking in Primary Healthcare: Realising Shared Aims in Patient Care.* London: Royal Pharmaceutical Society of Great Britain and the British Medical Association.

Spiegel, J.S., Spiegel, T.S. (1984) An Objective Examination of Multidisciplinary Patient Conference. *Journal of Medical Education* **59**(5), 436–438.

Spilsbury, K., Meyer, J. (2004) Use, misuse and non-use of health care assistants: understanding the work of healthcare assistants in a hospital setting. *Journal of Nursing Management* **12**(6), 411–418.

Stein, L. (1967) The Doctor–Nurse Game. *Archives of General Psychiatry* **18**(6), 699–703.

Stogdill, R.M. (1974) *Handbook of Leadership.* New York: Free Press.

Tope, R. (1996) *Integrated Interdisciplinary Learning Between the Health and Social Care Professions: A Feasibility Study.* Aldershot: Avebury.

United Cerebral Palsy, Nationally Organised Collaborative Comprehensive Service for Atypical Infants and Their Families (1976) *Staff Development Handbook: A Resource For The Transdisciplinary Process.* New York: United Cerebral Palsy Association.

Webb, A. (1986) Collaboration in planning: a prerequisite of community care? In: A. Webb and G. Wistow (eds) *Planning Needs and Scarcity, Essays on Personal Social Services.* London: Allen and Unwin.

William, R.A., Williams, C. (1982) Hospital social workers' and nurses' inter-professional perceptions and experiences. *Journal of Nursing Education* **21**(5), 16–21.

Wise, H., Bechard, R., Rubin, I., Kyte, A. (1974) *Making Health Care Teams.* USA: Ballinger.

Woodruf, G., McGoniegel, M.J. (1988) Early intervention team approaches. The transdisciplinary model. In: J.B Jordan, J.J Gallaghr, P.L Hutinger and M.B Karnes (eds) *Early Childhood Special Education.* Reston: Birth to Three Council for Exceptional Children.

Zwarenstein, M., Atkins, J., Barr, H., Hammick, M., Koppel, I., Reeves, S. (1999) A systematic review of interprofessional education. *Journal of Interprofessional Care* **13**(4), 417–424.

Zwarenstein, M., Reeves, S., Barr, H., Hammick, M., Koppel, I., Atkins, J. (2001) Interprofessional education: effects on professionals practice and health care outcomes (*Cochrane Review*). Oxford: The Cochrane Library, Issue 3.

2: Management of self, health service users and their families

Mandy Jones and Alison Warland

Embarking on a career as a healthcare professional provides a multitude of challenges to the newly qualified graduate. Having completed several years of training and gaining a broad spectrum of theoretical and clinical skills, the time then comes to action this accumulated knowledge as an independent, autonomous practitioner. However, not all the skills required to fulfil this role are a product of the classroom, but gained over time with practice experience when working.

The aims of this chapter are two-fold; firstly, to provide the reader with some concept and insight into the organisational and self-management skills necessary to become a successful healthcare professional, and secondly, to furnish the healthcare professional with the skills necessary to effectively manage service users and their families. As such, the information provided is drawn both from an evidence base and personal experience.

Professional practice

A profession is described as an occupation, vocation or career where specialized knowledge of a subject, field, or science is applied (Oxford English Dictionary, 1989). Healthcare professions are regulated by professional bodies, which act as a licensing authority for practitioners and enforce adherence to an ethical code of practice.

Professional codes of conduct and practice are multifactorial, covering aspects of direct patient contact, competence and professional development, multiprofessional liaison, ethical and personal behaviour (CSP, 2002; NMC, 2004; COT, 2005). By practising as a licensed healthcare professional, each individual has agreed to abide by these rules and regulations and is therefore accountable for their maintenance. Most healthcare professionals are conscientious and regularly audit and review their skills, in order to highlight areas of practice that require further training and development. However, some aspects of personal behaviour such as attitude, punctuality and appearance are less easily self-evaluated. In addition, most people have experienced a difficult situation within their personal life, which promotes a change of attitude, tolerance or demeanour that subsequently impacts on their professionalism (see Managing own emotions and maintaining professional boundaries). This may lead to a lack of focus, poor communication, misunderstanding or work becoming a reduced priority.

Self-management

The role of a healthcare professional extends beyond the pivotal focus of patient-centred practice and incorporates an abundance of non-clinical management, in particular of one's self! Effective self-management is essential to ensure efficient working with the minimal amount of stress. Self-management is, by definition, an individual learning process; however, early awareness and development of this skill is highly recommended.

Self-management refers to a collection of methods, techniques and strategies which can be employed to direct oneself to the achievement of specific objectives (Allen, 2001). Clinically, this may include the organisation and prioritisation of a patient caseload, effective time management, goal planning and setting, self-evaluation, continued professional development as well as the ability to manage one's own emotions and maintain professional boundaries.

Organisation and prioritisation of a caseload

The current healthcare environment requires healthcare professionals to manage the care of a rising number of patients, often with complex co-morbidity, with the same or an ever reducing number of staff. As such, the ability to work efficiently is being tested now more than ever. Although not ideal, it is a reality that not all referred patients will be reviewed and treated on a daily basis. In some cases, a patient viewed as a 'low priority' may only be seen once a week. Effective teamworking, including the delegation of appropriate patients to be managed by assistants, can maximise productivity. However, each healthcare professional must organise and prioritise their patient caseload, in order to identify which patients will be treated, and in what order, on any given day. Some flexibility may be necessary to incorporate both unplanned referrals and new admissions that may require urgent assessment and management.

In general, priority should be given to patients who are clinically unstable or those who may deteriorate without review and intervention. Second in priority are patients who remain vulnerable and must be reassessed, such as first and second day postoperative surgical patients or patients recently embarking on a course of medical management. Third are patients who are subacute or stable but still require input to gain full recovery or maximise independence and achieve hospital discharge. Finally there are patients who have stable chronic conditions for whom therapeutic intervention contributes to an on-going maintenance management programme.

Several situations may arise, which need to be considered when prioritising and formulating a patient caseload; some patients may be managed with reference to a specific clinical pathway or in accordance with a government derived framework (e.g., National Service Frameworks) which dictates therapeutic input at particular times during the recovery period. Many patients may require the combined input of more than one healthcare professional either from the same or an allied discipline; this necessitates careful liaison and time management. Critically ill or unstable patients may need to be reassessed throughout the day (Woodard and Jones, 2000), and often require lengthy and often unpredictable treatment periods.

Before organising and prioritising a caseload it is important to ensure all the necessary information is available to assist the healthcare professional to make an informed choice regarding the order of their patient list. Being knowledgeable can save time and effort; however, this may not always be possible as often several members of the multiprofessional team want to read the same set of patient notes, particularly if the patient is a new admission. Once familiarised with the caseload, if you remain unsure how to prioritorise the patients, discuss your thoughts with a line manager or a more experienced colleague who will be able to provide guidance.

Key points to prioritisation include:

▪ Read through patient caseload.
▪ Gather any additional information required.
▪ Identify urgency of patient's problems and rank appropriately.
▪ Make a case list and stick to it.
▪ Allocate slightly more time for each patient than anticipated.
▪ Factor in time for new or unexpected referrals.
▪ Anticipate an unmanageable caseload and either delegate or ask for help.
▪ Re-organise list throughout the day as clinical scenarios change.
▪ Make notes about each patient to assist prioritisation the following day.

Time management

> Good time management can be likened to a swan on a lake – calm, serene and controlled on the surface, but paddling like crazy underneath!

Time management is a rather ambiguous term, as it is not actually time which can be managed but rather our effective use of it (Allen, 2001). However, working within the healthcare environment rarely occurs in isolation; as a multiprofessional team member in a busy clinical environment (based either in the acute or community setting), a diversity of skills and abilities are required on a daily basis. As such, any one individual's ability to effectively manage their own time may be intrinsically linked with the abilities of other team members (Gorman, 1998). Often it is the interruption caused by an essential but unplanned liaison with colleagues or the arrival of a newly admitted acute patient which causes a shift in priorities and throws a carefully planned day out of balance. Therefore, in order to manage time efficiently and maximise professional effectiveness, strategies and plans need to be regularly re-evaluated and prioritorised accordingly (Hoover, 2007).

In order to start to develop individual time management skills, it is often a useful exercise to reflect on an average week within the workplace and identify the obstacles which have reduced effectiveness (Total Success website).

Common problems reducing productivity include (Total Success website):

- Interruption:
  - meetings;
  - unplanned discussion with other team members;
  - telephone calls;
  - visitors;
  - socializing.
- Indecision:
  - procrastination;
  - lack of preparation;
  - lack of expertise to deal with a situation;
  - unclear aims and objectives;
  - stress and fatigue.
- Communication issues:
  - unclear or poor communication.
- Poor planning:
  - lack of preparation;
  - lack of expertise;
  - poor evaluation of progress.
- Inadequate information:
  - poor communication;
  - poor preparation.
- Poor delegation:
  - keeping tasks which can be delegated;
  - inability to say 'no' to additional tasks.

Once personal obstacles have been identified, strategies to remove them can be implemented. Several categories fall under the general remit of being poorly prepared: lacking direction or information, expertise or training. Once acknowledged, these elements can be remedied with additional training and adequate planning. Every healthcare professional has an obligation in accordance with the code of professional conduct (CSP, 2002; COT, 2005) to be competent to perform interventional procedures. Therefore, any identified training needs must be discussed with a line manager and addressed as required. The newly qualified graduate must be confident in recognising their own clinical limitations when faced with treating a patient with a more complex or atypical presentation. Junior team members should always be encouraged to ask for support and advice from a senior colleague.

Unplanned interruptions provide the most difficult obstacle to resolve. An opportune discussion with a colleague about a patient's progress or management is an invaluable exercise; however, it may take considerable time and necessitate a reorganisation of the day's work. Try to keep impromptu meetings to a limited time scale. If a more detailed discussion is required, schedule a specific time when the issues can be raised in full without distraction. Try not to undertake an unrealistic amount of work in one day; trying to fit it all in will lead to poor quality work or the risk of missing an important issue.

Telephone calls can be a great drain on time so try to keep the conversation to a minimum and to the point (Hill, 2002). Make a brief note of the main points needed to be discussed (Total Success website) and direct the conversation appropriately. Allocate a specific time during the day to return phone calls, reply to email and maintain documentation.

Careful organisation and prioritisation of a patient caseload are essential components of time management, particularly for a new graduate as clinical work forms a large part of their professional responsibilities. Once the caseload has been organised, other activities must be factored in, such as meetings and in-service training. To maximise efficiency, before starting work each day, divide tasks into essential and non-essential, then draw up a list in order of importance (Hill, 2002; Hoover, 2007). Making a 'to do' list is an extremely useful tool, described by experts as one of the most effective time management tools (Hoover, 2007). Completion of each item is a valuable way to evaluate productivity and direct focus to items to be completed. The 'to do' list also acts as a reference tool, providing the user with an accurate measure of their committed time (Hoover, 2007). This is very useful when asked to undertake additional tasks, as any available time can be assessed at a glance. Regular re-evaluation of the list allows early identification of time management problems, giving colleagues warning that their assistance may be required. Equally, use spare time wisely by updating documentation or responding to correspondence; once these tasks are completed offer assistance to other members of the team. Regular effective communication within the team promotes efficient service delivery (Gorman, 1998).

Key points to time management include:

▓ Organise and prioritise patient caseload.
▓ Identify other tasks to be achieved:
  ● meetings;
  ● in-service training;
  ● professional liaison.

- Make a 'to do' list.
- Check off each item on completion.
- Re-evaluate list and reorganise regularly.
- Allow time for documentation.
- Allow time to respond to telephone calls and email.
- Monitor how you use your time and make conscious changes to your behaviour.
- Identify obstacles which reduce effectively.
- Aim to address issues within your control.
- Try to avoid unnecessary distraction.

Personal goal planning

As a healthcare professional, small personal goals may be set on a daily basis in order to juggle the management of a clinical case load, plus attending multiprofessional team meetings, liaison with colleagues, undertaking in-service training and fulfilling essential documentation. A goal is the purpose towards which you direct your actions (Hoover, 2007).

Self-evaluation and professional development

Most healthcare professionals undergo a formal appraisal with their line manager on a regular basis. This valuable exercise gives an opportunity for the appraisee to identify specific objectives that they would like to fulfil during that period of work. Training needs are highlighted and an appropriate list of targets is agreed (Gorman, 1998). However, more regular self-evaluation is an essential life-long learning skill which should be developed during training and continued throughout professional practice. This may be undertaken in many ways: using formal models of reflective practice (see Chapter 3), discussing clinical performance and competence with a senior colleague, or as an exercise to recognise areas for continued development. Identifying and analysing one's own strengths and weaknesses provides a basis on which to focus professional growth. Areas of strength can be consolidated and utilised, whilst weaknesses may be resolved with education, coaching or support. This ensures that healthcare professionals are competent to practise in accordance with professional regulation (CSP, 2002; NMC, 2004; COT, 2005).

Areas to consider for evaluation may fall under several categories:

- Professional development:
  - development of new clinical skills;
  - identification of training needs;
  - in-service training attendance;

- presentations delivered;
- development of managerial skills.
- Communication:
  - intraprofessional liaison;
  - multiprofessional liaison;
  - patient communication;
  - accurate documentation.
- Service development:
  - contribution to service delivery.
- Obstacles to progression:
  - identification of barriers to progression;
  - possible solutions.

Effective self-evaluation often promotes improved self-confidence. Knowing one's own areas of strength facilitates self-belief, which enables the healthcare professional to undertaken responsibilities without hesitation or doubt. Confidence and empowerment lead to increased assertiveness, effective and decisive action (Holden & Renshaw, 2002), ultimately promoting high-quality patient care.

Key points to self-evaluation:

- Make a list of your strengths.
- Build on your strengths.
- Analyse and admit to weaknesses.
- Recognise obstacles contributing to weaknesses.
- Identify opportunities to resolve obstacles.
- Find appropriate support to address areas of weakness.
- View self-evaluation as a positive process.

Managing own emotions and maintaining professional boundaries

While it may seem obvious that bringing emotional problems to work should be avoided, healthcare professionals must also learn to avoid taking work-related emotions home. Part of being a professional involves managing one's emotions, developing the ability to separate one's personal and working life and maintaining appropriate professional boundaries. Failure to do so can result in problems for both the healthcare professional and the service user. From the service user's point of view, it may result in an increase in emotional distress, impair relationships with family and friends and can encourage overdependence on the healthcare professional which may ultimately hinder rehabilitation. From the viewpoint of the healthcare professional, failure to maintain a work–life balance and becoming too emotionally involved may affect their personal life and relationships and lead to problems of emotional 'burn-out' (Buckman, 1992) and absence from work.

Stress levels may rise as a result of work-related emotional involvement, or from home stresses bought to work; both may impair clinical judgment and the ability to consistently provide service users with the highest level of care. In addition, maintenance of professional boundaries is recognised in standards of practice and rules of conduct for healthcare professionals (CSP, 2002; NMC, 2004; COT, 2005) and failure to comply could potentially result in disciplinary proceedings.

However, separating emotions from work situations is not always easy, for example, when caring for the terminally ill. Indeed, it is natural to feel empathy for patients, and this caring side to an individual's personality may be one of the main reasons for entering a healthcare profession in the first place. Moreover, it could be argued that it is these qualities that enable a healthcare professional to provide a high level of care. Nevertheless, for the reasons outlined above, it is important that the healthcare professional, while demonstrating caring and empathy, maintains a professional distance. This involves developing the ability to recognise when they are becoming too emotionally involved and developing strategies to deal with this.

In some clinical settings (for example in oncology, head injury or paediatrics), procedures may be in place for monitoring and alleviating staff stress. In other circumstances, stress may not be overtly apparent and it is often the healthcare professional's colleagues, family and friends who detect problems. Emotional over-involvement can be exhibited in a variety of ways, including working a disproportionate amount of unpaid overtime or contact with the patient out of working hours. Problems may also be detected through self-reflection, discussion with colleagues, following review of case notes, or through the mentoring and appraisal processes. Other signs may be indicative of emotional stress, such as sleeplessness, short temperedness or tearfulness. Once the problem has been recognised, strategies can be developed to enable the healthcare professional to address these issues and rectify the imbalance. These strategies vary but may include:

- informal discussion with colleagues (while maintaining patient confidentiality);
- more formal discussion with a colleague through mentoring, case review or 'buddying' system;
- team meetings, discussions and critical incidence evaluations;
- using reflection as a tool to analyse the situation;
- attendance at counselling or seeing an occupational psychologist;
- attending a support group (these groups are often available in situations where a high level of emotional stress is inherent, for example in a paediatric oncology unit);
- swapping patients with colleagues.

To conclude, emotional stress is inevitable in some situations. However the healthcare professional must learn to recognise and handle this efficiently and effectively in order to maintain professional boundaries and manage patients optimally.

Managing service users and their families

It is generally accepted that a key factor for successful rehabilitation is including service users (and where appropriate, their families and carers) in the management and rehabilitation process. In a nutshell, the key to this is through effective communication. However, this is not always easy, particularly when having to break bad news, when expectations of treatment are unrealistic or when a service user's (or their relatives' or carers') behaviour inhibits effective communication.

The next section of this chapter aims to address some of these issues by exploring:

- several causes of inappropriate behaviour and discussing potential management strategies that may be employed to deal with them;
- the management of unrealistic expectations of treatment;
- approaches to breaking bad news to patients and effectively managing the consequences.

Management of inappropriate behaviour

Inappropriate behaviour may occur in many different guises including:

- actual or threatened physical violence;
- threats and threatening gestures;
- verbal abuse;
- intentional damage to property;
- sexual or racial harassment;
- sexually inappropriate behaviour;
- inappropriate emotional attachment to the healthcare professional;
- stalking.

Actual or the threat of physical violence is of particular concern. Although the overall numbers of assaults has recently fallen, in 2006–2007 there were still 53 709 physical assaults against NHS staff with assaults on hospital-based staff, in particular, actually increasing (NHS SMS, 2008).

As well as the distress and potential damage caused to the healthcare professional, violence and threatened violence may also result in staff absence (and the associated financial costs), emotional distress or may even result in the healthcare professional leaving the NHS (DOH, 2006). Furthermore, patient care and healthcare delivery are adversely affected as staff take time to deal with such incidents. In response the government has introduced various strategies including the 'Zero tolerance campaign' as well as conflict resolution training for many frontline staff. However, it can be seen that violence is still a big problem for healthcare professionals, particularly for less experienced staff (Burns, 1993).

There are many causes of inappropriate behaviour. It is worth spending a few moments thinking about possible causes of this behaviour as this may hold the key to preventing it escalating. Causes include:

- frustration and boredom;
- fear;
- anger (for example about a situation or a diagnosis);
- brain damage (such as may occur with traumatic and hypoxic brain injury, as well as with some neurological conditions such as dementia);
- hypoxia and other causes of confusion;
- drug abuse and/or withdrawal;
- effect of medication;
- alcohol;
- hypo- or hyperglycaemia;
- mental health disorders.

While aggressive behaviour towards healthcare professionals is clearly unacceptable, in some circumstances, through considering causes of inappropriate behaviour, it can be anticipated and therefore better managed, perhaps even preventing escalation of a situation. For example, a patient who has spent the day fasting and anxiously awaiting planned surgery is unlikely to respond well when told their operation has been cancelled. Similarly, the patient who has taken time out of a busy schedule to attend an outpatient appointment is highly likely to be angered by an unexplained 2-hour wait. However, if the reasons for delays were explained (for example, the delay may have been caused by a patient emergency), and patients were informed as early as possible, the level of frustration, boredom and anger may be minimised.

It can also be understood that a parent whose child is being removed by social services is likely to be angry and distressed and may potentially exhibit aggressive behaviour. It might also be anticipated that a patient with brain damage might be aggressive or behave in a sexually inappropriate manner as a result of their injury. By anticipating such potential triggers the healthcare professional can identify steps to minimise aggression and protect him- or herself.

It is outside of the scope of this chapter to discuss management of potential violence in detail and readers should attend relevant training sessions, consult the appropriate NHS security management service publications (see Further reading) and local procedure and policy documents for more detailed information. However, in brief, such management might take the form of allowing the patient time to calm down, by not rushing the encounter, by discussing the situation with them and allowing them to voice their anger while making the person aware that their behaviour is unacceptable (Edwards, 2000; Brigden and Memon, 2004). Edwards (2000) also suggests that the healthcare professional maintains a relaxed body posture, maintains eye contact and addresses the patient by name. Since failure to manage one's own emotions and remain calm is likely to exacerbate the situation, the healthcare professional needs to ensure that they speak calmly and quietly. If necessary, hospital security or the police should be summoned for assistance.

Where potential inappropriate behaviour has been identified, risk assessments should be undertaken and necessary precautions and recommendations adhered to. Safety equipment such as a mobile phone or alarm buzzer should be available, and other members of staff should be available to help if necessary. The healthcare professional should have an exit strategy to remove them from the situation if necessary and staff working in the community ought to have clear checking in procedures (NHS SMS, 2005). Moreover, all staff must be conversant with local policies and be aware of security contact numbers (DOH, 2007). Following an incident it is essential that the healthcare professional reports the incident to the appropriate authority and that they undergo a suitable debriefing and period of reflection.

In summary inappropriate behaviour can take many different forms; it has many causes, but regardless of the cause remains unacceptable and should not be viewed as a part of the job or tolerated in any form. When dealing with potentially difficult situations, healthcare professionals should try to anticipate and prevent inappropriate behaviour where possible. However, when unable to prevent inappropriate behaviour, healthcare professionals should endeavour to prevent their emotions escalating the problem where possible. In addition, healthcare professionals should:

- be aware of ways of coping when they are unable to prevent the situation;
- be aware of how to summon help;
- know how to safely leave the area;
- know how to report the situation;
- report any incident;
- reflect and learn from any incident.

Managing unrealistic expectations

Conflict between healthcare professionals and service users may occur due to a mismatch in expectation of management or treatment outcome. When service user's expectations are unrealistic a number of problems may result, including dissatisfaction with the service they receive or dissatisfaction with the end result, a refusal to leave the hospital or be discharged, non-compliance, non-attendance, complaints against staff members, hostility and possible aggression (Desmond, 2003). The situation is further exacerbated when healthcare professionals force treatment goals or treatments on service users. This mismatch in expectation is a common situation and one which can often be reversed or avoided through appropriate discussion, communication and joint goal setting (Kersten, 2004; HPC, 2007).

When faced with an unrealistic patient, the temptation is to avoid having to deal with the issue, thus allowing the patient to continue in their unrealistic expectations. However, in the author's experience, failure to manage unrealistic expectations results in a delay in problem solving and ultimately hinders rehabilitation; it rarely results in the problem disappearing! As such the healthcare professional has a responsibility to the service user to be empathetic but honest and realistic regarding treatment outcomes.

Establishing the patient's understanding and expectation of their condition is often a good way to start, by asking questions such as 'What have you been told about your condition?', 'What do you understand by your diagnosis?' or 'What are your expectations of what I can do for you?' Such questions enable the healthcare professional to establish the service user's baseline knowledge. It allows correction of misconceptions and filling in any gaps in knowledge. Once this has been achieved, realistic goals identifying an aspired end-point in the individualised management plan can be agreed with the service user, as discussed below.

Goal setting

Treatment goals can require interdisciplinary or multidisciplinary input and are categorised as being either long or short term. In order to accomplish a long-term goal, several short-term ones must first be achieved. This provides an organised structure to the treatment plan, maintains a focus of treatment while outlining the attainable steps required to ultimately reach the long-term goal. Achievement of each short-term target, in turn, demonstrates the successful outcome of a treatment, objective progression associated with patient improvement and recovery or maintenance (Figure 2.1).

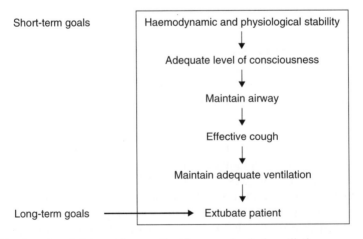

Figure 2.1 Treatment goals for weaning a patient from mechanical ventilation.

However, not all patient management follows this simple process. A patient may fail to respond to the treatment intervention or develop complications and co-morbidity leading to deterioration and decline. In addition, service users with deteriorating conditions may set goals aimed at maintaining function or quality of life or a goal aimed at minimising deterioration. Whatever sort of goals are set, it is vitally important to re-evaluate goals regularly to ensure they are appropriate, pertinent and achievable and that any treatment or management approach offered is suitable.

When writing a patient management plan, ensure the identified goals are realistic and specific. Document the proposed actions required to achieve each goal and how a successful outcome will be measured. A timeframe for completion of each goal should be set so adequate progression can be readily monitored and evaluated.

When a patient is unconscious the healthcare team may set goals on the patient's behalf. An example of appropriate medical and physiotherapy goals for a ventilated ITU patient are included in Figure 2.1. It should be remembered that wherever possible goal setting should be performed in conjunction with the service user (Kersten, 2004; HPC, 2007), as this is thought to increase treatment relevance and effectiveness (Baker et al, 2001; Kersten, 2004). However, problems occur when, in spite of education, open discussion and attempts to negotiate goals, healthcare professionals and service users differ in their expectations and cannot agree a goal. In such situations Hass (1993) recommends that as long as safety issues are addressed, the service users preferred goals are chosen. As goals should be regularly reviewed, in the author's experience, many service users will eventually realise when a goal is unrealistic and will adapt the goal accordingly. In spite of the difficulties in involving service users in the goal setting process, failure to do so can have serious repercussions on the rehabilitation process as illustrated by the case scenario in Box 2.1.

Key points to goal planning and setting:

■ Goal setting should be carried out in conjunction with the service user where possible.
■ Identify long-term goals.
■ Identify short-term goals required to reach long-term goal.
■ Identify individual steps necessary to achieve short-term goal.
■ Identify suitable outcome measures to measure progress.
■ Allocate a suitable timeframe to achieve and/review the goal.
■ Ensure goals are specific.
■ Ensure goals are achievable.
■ Re-evaluate goals regularly and update as required.

Breaking bad news and managing its consequences

When involved with patient care, most healthcare professionals will eventually be in the demanding situation of having to break bad news

Box 2.1 Scenario

The author was involved with the treatment of a young patient admitted with frequent falls and an inability to walk as a result of aggressively progressive multiple sclerosis. He had been deteriorating for some months and on examination was found to have profound weakness and a complete lack of sensation (including proprioception) in his lower limbs. It was felt unlikely that the patient would walk again and therefore the team decided that wheelchair mobility would be a safer and more realistic target for the patient to achieve.

Unfortunately no one had really involved the patient in this goal setting process! It was therefore unsurprising that he was uncompliant with attempts to teach him wheelchair skills. He frequently 'forgot' to attend therapy sessions. He complained the therapy staff didn't care, weren't treating him properly, were refusing to help him and accused them of not wanting him to walk again. He began to be openly hostile and verbally aggressive to staff. The situation culminated in the patient taking matters into his own hands and borrowing another patients' walking frame in an attempt to walk; a situation that ended with him falling and injuring both himself and the other patient.

The situation was resolved through education and open and honest discussion with the patient regarding his situation and prognosis. The team then sat down with the service user and together established joint goals that were agreeable to all parties. These included goals to achieve wheelchair independence as well as a goal surrounding independent walking. Although the healthcare team did not view the walking goal as being realistic, it was acknowledged that this was a goal that was very important to the patient and without its inclusion it was felt that the service user would continue to view the healthcare team as an enemy who didn't want him to walk and there was concern that in such a case he would remain uncompliant with treatment. The service user rapidly gained wheelchair independence and was discharged back to the community. Over time and through regular reviewing and resetting of goals he began to accept that he was unlikely to regain independent walking and eventually, at his own request, this was no longer set as a goal.

to the service user (or having to deal with the consequences of bad news broken by others). It is a task that is generally dreaded. However, no matter how strong the desire to avoid it, the responsibility must not be shrugged off, left for others to deal with or mishandled. Studies have demonstrated that a patient's ability to cope with bad news is linked with how the news was broken (Fallowfield, 1993), yet it is a subject that is rarely covered in training (Buckman, 1992; Rabow and McPhee, 2000; Farrell, 2002).

To start with, it is worth taking a few moments to consider what constitutes bad news. It is often thought of in the context of breaking news about death and dying or a life-changing diagnosis; for example news regarding diagnosing a child with ADHD, or informing the stroke patient that you think it is unlikely they will walk or talk again or gain functional use of their arm. While these situations are clearly ones of bad news, it is not the complete picture and news that a patient perceives as 'devastating' or 'bad' can be subtle and not always obvious to the healthcare professional. For example the news of a pregnancy may be felt by a healthcare professional to be cause for celebration. However, if this pregnancy was not planned or wished for it may be a devastating diagnosis for a patient. The patient who presented with a painful foot may be distraught to learn that the soft tissue injury you diagnose (although a short-term injury) will prevent him participating in a particular sport and missing the longed for competition he has been working hard for. Conversely, a patient presenting with neurological problems consistent with multiple sclerosis, may be relieved to discover that their symptoms are not due to the cancer they feared. The list is extensive and beyond the scope of this chapter to discuss, however, healthcare professionals need to be vigilant with their communication with patients and remember that what is perceived as bad news varies vastly between individuals.

Different diagnoses, individual personalities and individual situations mean that there is no one prescriptive method of breaking bad news. Healthcare professionals whose role regularly involves breaking bad news should consider further study of this demanding and complex area; however some basic guidelines may be useful to consider.

Where possible, the healthcare professional should thoroughly prepare for the interview (Buckman, 1992; DOH, 2003). The environment in which the news is to be broken should be considered and when necessary a private room should be booked, to limit noise and interruptions. If possible bleeps, telephones and pagers should be turned off or diverted. The healthcare professional may wish to consider having another member of staff or a member of the patient's family to support the patient and, on a practical note, a box of paper handkerchiefs may be useful.

Ideally the healthcare professional should ensure they have time to break the news appropriately and to deal with the consequences, allowing the service user an opportunity to vent their emotions and ask questions. In reality, finding adequate time may be difficult, but the healthcare professional must never appear to rush the situation. When time is limited, it is recommended that the service user is informed as such, and clearly told when you will return, giving the patient a suitable timeline. When breaking bad news, if possible, the healthcare professional should sit down, preferably close to the service user so, if appropriate, the healthcare professional can offer support through touch (Buckman, 1992). The healthcare professional should employ open body language and speak gently but clearly.

In some instances, service users may be aware that bad news is likely. This may occur following assessment, or if the results of a procedure or investigation are available. In this instance, the service user may ask you about their condition before you have considered how to discuss it. Conversely, the service user may not be prepared for the news and may find it difficult to cope.

In either situation it is useful to establish what the service user understands about their condition and prognosis and how much they wish to know about it. Questions such as: 'What have you been told about your condition?' or 'What do you understand about the diagnosis?' can be useful to help ascertain a patient's understanding. Buckman (1992) suggests identifying how much a patient wishes to know about their condition and subsequent management by asking them directly. Phrases such as 'Should the news turn out to be bad, do you wish me to tell you about this?', 'Would you prefer me to just discuss treatment options with you?' or 'Would you prefer that I discussed this with you or with someone else?' may be useful. Once this has been established the healthcare professional can then move on to actually breaking the news.

Before actually delivering bad news it is valuable to identify what phrases and words to use, or even write down a script in preparation (Rabow and McPhee, 2000) or mentally rehearse the discussion (DOH, 2003). Avoid use of medical jargon and words that can be misinterpreted. The author will never forget using the term 'cancer' to a lady with advanced breast cancer only to be told 'No dear, I don't have *cancer*. The doctor told me it was just a *tumour*. I thought it was cancer too. I'm so relieved!'

When delivering bad news try to be honest and direct. Phrases such as 'I'm sorry to have to tell you but. . .' or 'Unfortunately I have bad news' prepare the patient for what is to follow. Owens (1994) describes the need for a balance between optimism and pessimism when delivering bad news, and while remaining realistic it is important to provide reassurance when possible. This can be a fine balancing act and one which requires considerable tact, knowledge and skill. It may appear very obvious but it is worthwhile reiterating that the healthcare professional should be fully conversant with an individual's personal and medical history, facts about the service user's problems as well as a thorough understanding of any management and treatment options. If a question is asked that the healthcare professional cannot answer, she should admit this and inform the patient that she will provide the information as soon as possible (Buckman 1992). After delivering the news it is useful to check what the patient has understood. Providing the patient with written materials to support what has been discussed is often useful.

After breaking bad news and outlining management or treatment options, the healthcare professional should ascertain the service user's concerns and feelings and develop what Buckman (1992) refers to as a 'shopping list' of needs to be addressed and discussed. In practice this can be achieved through asking questions such as 'What are you most concerned about?' or simply 'What questions do you have for me?', as well as being vigilant to the service user's body language or 'throwaway' comments. In addition, as well as arranging a follow-up meeting when appropriate, the service user can be referred on to other agencies, e.g. counselling, the chaplaincy service or to a relevant support group.

Finally, breaking bad news properly can be extremely stressful and healthcare professionals should be aware of the effects of this on their own emotional state and take measures to ensure their own emotional well-being.

In summary, when breaking bad news healthcare professionals should:

- know the facts and prepare (consider making a script);
- consider the setting;
- ensure adequate time to break the news and deal with the consequences;
- ensure body language is appropriate;
- find out what patient knows/understands about their condition or situation;
- find out what the patient wants to know about their condition;
- admit when an answer is unknown and when possible find out the answer or refer the service user to an appropriate individual;
- try to find a balance between optimism and pessimism;
- ensure that communication is direct and honest;
- listen carefully, especially to anxieties and to what is not being verbalised;
- reassure where possible;
- follow up and refer onward as appropriate;
- deal effectively with own emotions.

Conclusion

During their career, the healthcare professional acquires a multitude of skills to effectively manage service users and their families and carers. Many of these are founded during undergraduate education and consolidated with clinical practice. However, other skills can only be developed through experience, reflection, self-awareness and on-going education. Early awareness and development of organisational and self-management skills equip the healthcare professional with expertise to efficiently provide optimal healthcare. Moreover, advancement and understanding of the service user's situation or experiences of care may prove essential to promote cohesive rehabilitation and ultimately an effective outcome.

Further reading

Breaking bad news

Buckman R (1992) How To Break Bad News. London: Pan Macmillan.

DOH (2003) Dept of Health, Social Services and Public Safety. Breaking Bad News Regional guidelines. Northern Ireland. http://www.dhsspsni.gov.uk/publications/2003/breaking_bad_news.pdf

http://www.breakingbadnews.co.uk/

Managing violent behaviour

NHS Security Management Service website has many useful publications and links. http://www.cfsms.nhs.uk/pubs/sms.gen.pubs.html

References

Allen, D. (2001) *Getting Things Done: The Art of Stress-Free Productivity*. New York: Penguin Putnam.

Baker, S., Marshak, H., Rice, G., Zimmerman, G. (2001) Patient participation in physical therapy goal setting. *Physical Therapy* **81**(5), 1118–1126.

Brigden, D., Memon, M. (2004) Dealing with aggressive patients. Occasional Paper, *Mersey Deanery Education Matters* Sheet 19.

http://www.merseydeanery.nhs.uk/graphics/File/Courses%20&%20Resources/Education%20Publications/Ed_Matters/Ed-no19.pdf (Accessed March 2008).

Buckman, R. (1992) *How To Break Bad News*. London: Pan Macmillan.

Burns, J. (1993) Working with Potential violence. In: R. Bayne and P. Nicolson (eds) *Counselling and Psychology for Health Professionals*. London: Chapman and Hall, pp. 51–56.

COT (2005) *Rules of Professional Conduct*. London: COT.

CSP (2002) *Rules of Professional Conduct*. London: CSP.

Desmond, J. (2003) *Managing Patient's Expectations*. 3(1) www.healthcarecollaborator.com (Accessed February 2008).

DOH (2003) Dept of Health, Social Services and Public Safety. *Breaking Bad News*. Regional guidelines. Northern Ireland. http://www.dhsspsni.gov.uk/publications/2003/breaking_bad_news.pdf. (Accessed March 2008).

DOH (2006) *Tackling Nuisance or Disturbance Behaviour on NHS Premises: A Paper for Consultation*. London: DOH.

DOH (2007) *National Task Force on Violence: Employee Checklist*. London: DOH.

DOH. National Service Frameworks. http://www.dh.gov.uk/en/Policyandguidance/Healthandsocialcaretopics/DH_4070951 (Accessed 29th October 2007).

Edwards, W. (2000) *Management of Aggressive Patients*. www.ukppg.org.uk/01-06-dumphries-managing-aggressive-patients.rtf (Accessed April 2008).

Fallowfield, L. (1993) Giving sad and bad news. *Lancet* **341**, 476–478.

Farrell, M. (2002) Breaking bad news. In: T. Shaw and K. Sanders (eds) *Foundation of Nursing Studies Dissemination Series* **1**(2), 1–4.

Gorman, P. (1998) *Managing Multi-disciplinary Teams in the NHS*. London: Open University Press.

Hass, J. (1993) Ethical considerations of goal setting for patient care in rehabilitation medicine. *American Journal of Physical Medicine and Rehabilitation* **72**, 228–232.

Holden, R., Renshaw, B. (2002) Leadership Career Centre. Newsletter update May 3rd http://www.leadershipcareercenter.com/articles/20020503-newsletter.doc (Accessed 7th December 2007).

Hoover, J. (2007) *Best Practices: Time Management*. New York: Harper Collins.

HPC (2007) *Standards of Proficiency*. London: HPC.

Kersten, P. (2004) Principles of physiotherapy assessment and outcome measures. In: M. Stokes (ed) *Physical Management in Neurological Rehabilitation*, 2nd edn. London: Elsevier Mosby.

NHS SMS (2005) *Not Alone: A Guide for the Better Protection of Lone Workers in the NHS*. London: NHS SMS.

NHS SMS (2008) http://www.cfsms.nhs.uk/doc/press.release/ycot_launches_kent_08.pdf. (Accessed May 2008).

NMC (2004) The *NMC code of Professional conduct: performance and ethics standards*. 07.04. London: NWC.

Owens, P. (1994) Palliative care. In: P. Owens, J. Carrier and J. Horder (eds) *Interprofessional Issues in Community and Primary Health Care*. Wiltshire: Palgrave Macmillan, pp. 165–183.

Oxford English Dictionary (1989) Second edition. Oxford: Oxford University Press.

Rabow, M., McPhee, S. (2000) Beyond breaking bad news: helping patients who suffer. *Student BMJ* **8**, 65–67.

Total Success. http://www.totalsuccess.co.uk/timemanagementskills.htm. (Accessed 29th October 2007).

Woodard, F., Jones, M. (2000) Intensive care for the critically ill adult. In: J.A. Pryor and S.A. Prasad (eds) *Physiotherapy for Respiratory and Cardiac Problems. 1 Adults & Paediatrics*, 3rd edn. London: Churchill Livingston.

3: Reflection and professional practice

Alison Blank

The term reflective practice is used in many different walks of professional life, including teaching at all levels: from primary to post graduate, mainstream and special needs; nursing within mental health, learning disabilities and general nursing; social work; physiotherapy; counselling and occupational therapy. Reflective practice is a fundamental component of continued professional development, which is required by all regulatory bodies of healthcare professions in order to retain registration (see Chapter 10). Although an occupational therapist by training, I have attempted to present a generic overview of reflective practice which will be useful irrespective of the reader's individual professional identity and place of employment. There is however an emphasis upon the professions of physiotherapy and occupational therapy.

Kramer (1974) and Schmalenberg and Kramer (1976) described 'reality shock' as the dissonance experienced by qualified nurses on comparing placement education with the reality of clinical practice and its associated stress and crisis of confidence. The early months of a professional life may be a crucial time for using reflection on practice as a way of adjusting to life as a qualified healthcare professional and enhancing the development of a professional identity. However, it should be noted that reflective practice is a broad concept and is not without its critics; moreover there is no universally accepted definition. Ghaye and Ghaye (1998) asked 50 experienced teachers what they understood by reflective practice. Their answers ranged from somewhat negative interpretations such as 'navel gazing' and 'the latest bandwagon', to more positive perspectives, such as 'learning from experience', 'gaining confidence in your work' and 'personal growth'.

Despite the absence of a single definition of reflective practice, it may be useful to consider two accepted definitions. Creek (1997:132) states 'the process of observation, interpretation, and decision making during intervention is called reflective practice'. Within the physiotherapy profession the generally accepted definition provided by Boud et al (1985:19) is 'a generic term for those intellectual and affective activities in which individuals engage to explore their experiences in order to lead to new understandings and appreciations'. However the definitions and interpretation given above imply a relatively narrow focus upon oneself and one's own practice. Therefore, my own interpretation of these definitions, and the one on which this chapter is based, is that reflective practice is a means by which practitioners can develop greater levels of self-awareness about themselves as practitioners and as people. This in turn can lead to opportunities for professional development and personal growth. Bolton (2001) considers the social and political contexts of reflective practice and argues that to be fully and usefully reflective we need to look beyond ourselves to the social and political environments within which our practice is located. However, this may be a level of reflective practice to which we can aspire but may be difficult for newly qualified practitioners to achieve, although the importance of the continued development of reflective practice skills throughout one's career as a healthcare professional must be stressed.

The advent of clinical governance and the need for continuing professional development (CPD) introduced other strategic ways in which reflective practice could be used. Modernisation and Agenda for Change (DOH, 2004) introduced preceptorship which aims to provide consistency across clinical areas, through adequate support and supervision of newly qualified staff. Preceptorship may also facilitate the transition from learner to practitioner by advocating and developing reflective practice skills. However, these strategic uses of reflective practice may have contributed to a negative perspective (Ghaye & Ghaye, 1998). It is easy to see how reflective practice and supervision might be viewed as a way of managers 'checking up' on staff and not as a tool to facilitate professional development and growth. Mackintosh (1998) suggests that there are unproven benefits to the nursing profession and that there is uncertainty for its implementation in practice. Gilbert (2001), another critic of reflective practice, argues that reflective practice can be seen as a form of 'surveillance' and is critical of its association and links with clinical supervision. However, Clouder and Sellars (2004) disagree; they acknowledge that we are all subject to surveillance one way or another and argue that supervision and surveillance become more ethical if presented and developed through reflective practice. Johns (1995) suggests that it enables professionals to define contradictions between their actual practice and desired practice as well as enhancing clinical expertise which in turn improves practice.

As a concept reflective practice can seem quite complex and rather esoteric. There is not a 'one size fits all' approach to practice which will magically solve all your problems and enable you to grow as a professional. Indeed, becoming an effective reflective practitioner is something which takes work, practice and commitment. Therefore the primary aim of this chapter is to demystify reflective practice, critically examine its importance and outline its advantages and disadvantages in professional practice. Secondarily, the chapter aims to encourage the reader to think about his or her own views and experiences of reflective practice and how to continue to utilise this valuable skill.

Using reflection in practice

Implicit in Creek's (1997) definition are differences between reflection *on* practice and reflection *in* practice. Bolton (2001:15) describes the reflection *in* practice as 'the hawk in your mind constantly circling over your head watching and advising you on your actions – while you are practising'. Reflection *on* practice is the post hoc thinking, writing and discussing what occurred after the event, which links with the development of clinical reasoning (Mattingly & Fleming, 1994). Reflection in action is a skill which develops with practice and experience and improves with confidence, described by Mattingly and Fleming (1994) as an aspect of the expert practitioner. However, for the novice practitioner there is much to be learned from focusing on post hoc reflection on practice. In order to learn from our practice we must focus on the whole experience and seek to understand the significance within it. It is this ability to extract meaning from experiences that we need to consolidate and develop in order to influence future practice. In the Casson Memorial lecture to the College of Occupational Therapists annual conference, Taylor (2007) warned that it is not enough just to have experiences in order to learn, but effective reflection upon that experience is a crucial part of the process. Gibbs (1988) supports this view stating that all too often the reflective step in the learning cycle is lost. Very often even experienced practitioners will jump from a superficial account of what happened to premature plans about what to do next. This may be due to pressure of time and lack of experience in and commitment to reflection. Furthermore 'doing' something may often be easier than staying with and reflecting on uncomfortable feelings and experiences.

Why is reflective practice important?

There is still limited evidence to demonstrate empirically that reflective practice is effective. However, there is evidence that expertise does not derive from the application of rules and procedures, but instead, professional wisdom stems from highly developed intuition which can be difficult to articulate but can be demonstrated in practice (Gould, 1996). Bolton (2001) suggests that reflective practice can enable us to think about our own decision-making processes, help us to be constructively critical of relationships with our colleagues, help to identify knowledge and skills deficits and identify learning needs and assist us in facing difficult and painful clinical encounters. It is also a useful tool in supervisory relationships, such as peer supervision as a group or part of a pair, a student/educator relationship, a mentor/preceptor relationship or as part of the reflexive aspect of the research process.

Kolb (1984) identified reflection as a key stage in the learning cycle. He suggests that effective reflective practice may be a valuable tool in learning, which may be applicable to all sorts of areas of practice and in a multitude of different formats. Furthermore, reflective practice can be an important way to begin to integrate theory with practice, to bridge the gap which is often a challenge to newly qualified practitioners. Donaghy and Morss (2000, 2007) argue that it is important to move away from a reflective approach which focuses on individual practitioners' beliefs, attitudes and values and adopt an approach which encompasses systematic critical enquiry, problem solving and clinical reasoning. The development of a style of reflective practice which encompasses both aspects, a focus on therapist attitudes and a focus on critical enquiry, may provide the practitioner with a set of skills which can be applied to any situation. Gard et al (2000) suggest that, although physiotherapists have an awareness of their patients' underlying emotions, they often do not respond to this in treatment, but favour responses on an intellectual level. In their study, Gard et al (2000) found it was important to promote verbal expressions of emotion in treatment situations, as this can initiate a reflective process in practitioners with immediate understanding of the interaction.

As each of us grows and develops in our clinical role, an individual understanding of what reflective practice means will influence and shape our own reflective style. I want to develop an argument for reflective practice as an art, employed creatively, in different ways by individual practitioners but ultimately fulfilling the same purpose. This notion is supported by other writers, including Bleakley (1999) and Winter (1999), who consider the 'artistry' of reflective practice.

Reflective practice is not easy; it can be challenging, demanding and ultimately quite trying. It can invoke feelings which are uncomfortable, exposing and frustrating; however, striving to integrate it into practice is essential rather than an optional extra.

Many practitioners claim to be already practising reflectively; indeed, most of us do recapture and evaluate our experiences on a regular basis. Donald Schon (1991), acknowledged by many to be one of the pioneers of reflective practice, maintains that there are several possible models of reflection including conversations in the head, informal conversations with colleagues, written records, discussions with colleagues acting as 'critical friends', as well as more formal arrangements for supervision and appraisal. Although, not always popular, journal writing is another option (Bolton, 2001). Reflective diaries work for some people although there is divided opinion about their usefulness. Some researchers feel they dwell too much on the descriptive and observational stages of reflection and lack interpretation and analysis. My own feeling is that writing about something can be a good starting point, and is a habit which may be useful later on in the form of research field notes. The key is to identify the optimal approach that works for each individual.

Strands of reflection

It is important that you choose the reflective practice aid that best suits your own individual learning styles and needs. Fish et al (1991) describe four strands of reflection – factual, retrospective, substratum and connective. These are progressive stages of the reflective process that can be applied to any situation. A case study is provided to illustrate this process (Box 3.1). The first strand, the factual strand, is simply telling the story. It is primarily descriptive and is the first step towards practising reflectively; it is not exploring what happened in any depth rather just recounting a series of events. It is possible that some practitioners, especially novices, do not progress any further beyond this stage. However,

---

Box 3.1 Case example, Molly's mother

I first met Molly when she was due to be discharged from the inpatient unit of a local mental health unit following a short admission with a suspected psychotic episode. She was referred to the Community Mental Health Team in which I was working at the time. Molly was a young woman of 20 years who lived with her mother. She was the youngest child, having three older brothers who had all left home. Molly did reasonably well at school and went on to college to do computer studies. It was while she was at college that she became mentally unwell. She began neglecting her personal care, sleeping a lot, thought people were talking about her and so stopped attending college. She felt afraid of people and spent time sitting apparently not doing anything. Concerned, her mother encouraged her to consult their GP who referred Molly to a psychiatrist. I met Molly's mother on a number of occasions, usually at the 6-monthly reviews with her psychiatrist to which she always accompanied her daughter. On these occasions Molly's mother always seemed very anxious and although the psychiatrist and I tried our best to make the meetings as informal and friendly as possible, we all found them very difficult.

During the time I was working with Molly I was aware that her mother found the situation quite difficult but despite attempts to engage her in conversation she remained quite aloof and I felt we had an uneasy relationship. Then something happened which changed this. I was aware of the importance of work for people with mental health problems and thought Molly might want to discuss this option, so I wrote to her to suggest we meet to talk about a work assessment. The day the letter arrived I received a phone call from Molly's mother who was extremely angry and upset that I seemed to be suggesting that Molly should be thinking about going back to work. During the conversation she poured out all her anger and grief about what had happened to her daughter, her dislike of the review meetings and her worries about what would happen to Molly when she was no longer around to look after her.

It was hard to be on the receiving end of so much anger and pain, so as soon as possible I made time to talk with my supervisor about the phone call. In the factual strand of our reflective session I recounted the narrative of the story.

I presented the facts and details for my supervisor so that we could both see and understand what we were to discuss. Sometimes going over the sequence of events is in itself helpful, particularly if the incident has been in any way traumatic. However, it is not always the dramatic that needs reflecting on, we can learn much by reflecting deeply on the ordinary and everyday aspects of our work. In the second strand, the retrospective strand, my supervisor and I began to look for patterns and connections. I knew from previous work in child and family services that working with families is a skilled job which can be difficult. Parents are naturally protective of their children even when in adulthood like Molly; I know from my own experiences as a parent of a young adult what a difficult and challenging task it can be. In this strand we began to draw together my previous personal and professional experiences, to try and understand the conversation with Molly's mother more clearly and what I could learn from it.

The substratum strand requires close examination of one's own values and beliefs. One of mine is around client-centred practice and respecting Molly as an adult individual, even though I knew from my contact with the family that this was not really how they related. Molly's mother tended to treat her as if she were a younger child, which was challenged by my writing directly to Molly. This may have been what upset her mother. Whatever the reason, I was able to see that my values and thus the way I acted (by writing to Molly) were at odds with my previous interaction with this family. In addition as an occupational therapist I knew the importance of work for individuals with mental illness and wanted to include this on the agenda for my interventions with Molly. Perhaps if I was being truly client-centred I should have waited for this to come from Molly herself?

Finally, in the connective strand attempts are made to draw all the reflective strands together, to process what has been learnt and to plan for future action. In this case there was a meeting between Molly, her mother, the psychiatrist and myself to discuss the issues that had been raised. Having been already able to voice and register her distress, Molly's mother appeared more relaxed in the discussions that followed. We also agreed that future meetings would take place at the family home and that there was no need for the consultant to attend. In this way we made the contact between Molly's family and the mental health services less formal and thus more acceptable to Molly's mother. From this situation I learnt the need for a sensitive approach to clients' families and the timing of interventions. Maybe with hindsight I would not have acted any differently but it was important to have reviewed the situation to understand it more fully.

it is important to learn to build upon the strands to maximise the learning experience. Some practitioners find writing the story down a useful strategy, as writing slows down the thinking process and provides a record for discussion and later reflection (Field, personal communication). It is important to allow time to develop your reflective skills; like anything, they will improve with practice. You cannot apply a reflective approach to everything so be selective and remember you can learn as much from the ordinary as from the extraordinary.

There are a number of models of reflective practice, the one developed by Fish et al (1991) using four reflective strands, has already been

Box 3.2 Example of Gibbs' model in practice

1. What happened? I met Paul and Brian in a café in their local town. We found a quiet table, sat with our drinks and discussed a letter and information sheet that I drafted to invite people to take part in a research project. Paul and Brian had lots of useful comments and Paul had brought along a redraft that he had already done.
2. How was I feeling? This was my third meeting with Paul (but first with Brian) so I was feeling more confident and more relaxed. I was aware of feeling more able to leave behind my therapist role and take on that of a researcher working collaboratively. I was also aware of the different power relationships – I was asking them to help me.
3. Evaluation. This was a really useful meeting. Both Paul and Brian contributed ideas and thoughts that were genuinely helpful to me. I thought I picked up on some tensions between them related to a user group to which they both belong.
4. Analysis. Having coffee helped add to the meeting's informality which I think made us all feel quite relaxed. Brian was able to catch up with issues Paul and I had discussed in our previous meetings.
5. Conclusion. This meeting marked the end of the first round of consultation with the user panel. The initial paperwork I needed was complete and has been fully approved by the mental health service user panel. I felt that there had been meaningful (as opposed to tokenistic) mental health service user involvement in this stage of the study.
6. Action. After my next academic supervision, I will feed back to the panel to let them know the next stage. I will use this reflection to analyse in more detail the user involvement experience. I will arrange for the user panel to meet again in a few months to continue to invest in those relationships and keep the momentum going.

described. Gibbs (1988) provides another which is very useful. It is similar to that of Fish but utilises headings which may be easier to comprehend. When using the model by Gibbs (1998), firstly describe what happened – tell the story. Secondly, describe how it made you feel, then, thirdly, attempt to evaluate the experience. Follow this with an analysis, a conclusion and finally a plan for action. In the following case study, Gibbs' (1988) model has been applied to a brief reflection on a meeting between myself and two mental health services users, who are part of a group advising me on a research project (Box 3.2).

A good supervisor with whom you have an honest and trusting relationship will be an invaluable aid to your development as a reflective practitioner. When working in clinical practice the best supervisors were often the ones I was allowed to choose for myself. Very often these days, allocated supervisors are also your line manager which can make it difficult to be truly honest about aspects of your practice about which you are unsure. Like any relationship, a supervisory one takes work and commitment so it is important to invest in your relationship with your supervisor. Prioritising supervision is one way of doing this

> **Box 3.3** Cue questions
>
> ■ Did you make any assumptions?
> ■ Do you think the patient sees the problem differently?
> ■ Are all of the problems physiotherapy problems?
> ■ Are these the problems you would expect?
> ■ What other factors may be present?
>
> Donaghy and Morss (2000)

but all too often with busy clinical schedules it can be the first thing to be cancelled to create space in a packed diary. Try very hard not to do this, as you will ultimately be a better more thoughtful and self-aware clinician if you make good use of regular supervision.

Reflection as part of a group has been advocated by some as having the power to change practice. *Psychosis Revisited* (Bassett et al, 2007) is a two-day workshop for mental health workers, which provides a space for teams who work with people experiencing psychosis to stand back and reflect on their practice. The workshop ends with an action planning session where teams can formulate plans to make changes to the ways they work and relate to each other and their clients. Donaghy and Morss (2000), researchers in physiotherapy, advocate what they term guided reflection. They found that this approach enabled students and novice practitioners to develop deeper reflective skills. This approach makes use of cue questions under the guidance of an experienced reflective practitioner. Some examples of these cue questions are given in Box 3.3.

Reflective practice does not have to be complicated. It is a skill to be developed throughout your professional life. Start small by committing time and energy to it by prioritising supervision, using a reflective diary and fostering relationships with people with whom you can talk reflectively about your work. Consider using a model that is easy to use – experiment with the ones included here, or look at the website of your relevant professional body where you will find additional useful information. Your ability to be a reflective practitioner will develop with practice and you will become a more mature, effective and fulfilled practitioner, who is able to make a valuable and valid contribution to patient care as a result.

References

Bassett, T. Hayward, M. Chandler, R., Blank, A. (2007) *Psychosis Revisited*, 2nd edn. Brighton: Pavilion.

Bleakley, A. (1999) From reflective practice to holistic reflexivity. *Studies in Higher Education* **24**(3), 215–330.

Bolton, G. (2001) *Reflective Practice. Writing and Professional Development*. London: Sage.

Boud, D., Keogh, R., Walker, D. (1985) Promoting reflection in professional courses: the challenges of context. *Studies in Higher Education* **23**(2), 191–206.

Clouder, L., Sellars, J. (2004) Reflective practice and clinical supervision: an interprofessional perspective. *Journal of Advanced Nursing* **46**(3), 262–269.

Creek, J. (1997) Treatment planning and implementation. In: J. Creek (ed) *Occupational Therapy and Mental Health*, 2nd edn. London: Churchill Livingstone.

Department of Health (2004) *NHS Knowledge and Skills Framework (NHS KSF) and the Development Review Process*. London: The Stationery Office.

Donaghy, M., Morss, K. (2000) Guided reflection: a framework to facilitate and assess reflective practice within the discipline of physiotherapy. *Physiotherapy Theory and Practice* **16**(1), 3–14.

Donaghy, M., Morss, K. (2007) An evaluation of a framework for facilitating and assessing physiotherapy students' reflection on practice. *Physiotherapy Theory & Practice* **23**(2), 83–94.

Fish, D., Twinn, S., Purr, B. (1991) *Promoting Reflection: Improving the Supervision of Practice in Health Visiting and Initial Teacher Training*. Twickenham: West London Institute.

Gard, G., Gyllenstan, A.L., Salford, E., Ekdahl, C. (2000) Physical therapists' emotional expressions in interviews about factors important for interaction with patients. *Physiotherapy* **86**(5), 229–240.

Ghaye, A., Ghaye, K. (1998) *Teaching and Learning through Critical Reflective Practice*. London: David Fulton.

Gibbs, G. (1988) *Learning by Doing*. London: Further Education Unit.

Gilbert, T. (2001) Reflective practice and clinical supervision: meticulous rituals of the confessional. *Journal of Advanced Nursing* **36**(2), 199–205.

Gould, N. (1996) Introduction. In: N. Gould and I. Taylor (eds) *Reflective Learning for Social Work: Research, Theory and Practice*. Aldershot: Arena.

Johns, C. (1995) The value of reflective practice for nursing. *Journal of Clinical Practice* **4**(1), 23–30.

Kramer, M. (1974) *Reality Shock: Why Nurses Leave Nursing*. St. Louis MO: Mosby.

Kolb, D.A. (1984) *Experiential Learning*. London: Prentice Hall.

Mattingly, C., Fleming, M. (1994) *Clinical Reasoning: Forms of Inquiry in a Therapeutic Practice*. Philadelphia: F.A. Davis.

Mackintosh, C. (1998) Reflection a flawed strategy for the nursing profession. *Nursing Education Today* **18**(7), 553–557.

Schmalenberg, C.E., Kramer, M. (1976) Dreams and reality: where do they meet? *Journal of Nursing Administration* **6**(5), 35–43.

Schon, D. (1991) *The Reflective Practitioner. How Professionals Think in Action*, 2nd edn. Aldershot: Arena.

Taylor, M.C. (2007) Casson Memorial Lecture 2007: Diversity amongst occupational therapists – Rhetoric or Reality? *British Journal of Occupational Therapy* **70**(7), 276–283.

Winter, R. (1999) *Learning from Experience*. Lewes: Falmer.

4: Challenges of client-centred practice in professional practice

Thelma Sumsion

Client-centred practice now forms the basis for interventions in many professions. Both professional associations and client groups have identified the importance of treating people as individuals rather than clones within a large system (Bibyk et al, 1999; CAOT, 2002; COT, 2005). However, it is important for the health professional to recognise that the successful application of this approach entails a very complicated process. Using the words 'client-centred' when addressing clients, or incorporating these words into mission statements, does not mean that the relevant concepts are actually being applied. Therefore, this chapter endeavours to assist emerging health professionals to determine their personal working definition of client-centred practice, focus on some of the key challenges when attempting to apply this approach, and consider some strategies for facilitating success.

Defining client-centred practice

The first step in the successful application of a client-centred approach is to understand the concepts inherent within it and focus on a definition that has personal meaning. There is a range of definitions in the literature and authors from many disciplines have suggested components of this approach or fuller definitions that are important to consider (Gillespie et al, 2004; Zandbelt et al, 2006). A clear statement within dentistry is that this approach to practice simply means that 'the majority of your practice modalities should be designed to serve the patient first' (Brown, 2001:10). A medical author suggests that it is important to know patients as people in addition to diagnosing their illness (Epstein, 2000). Others have suggested that this approach is synonymous with many important and relevant concepts, which will be discussed in a later section, including negotiation, sharing decision making and facilitating client participation in planning interventions (Redfern et al, 2006).

Canadian occupational therapists have accepted the importance of a client-centred approach since the early 1980s. Their views of and approach to this concept have continued to develop over the intervening years. One accepted definition that has enhanced that process was outlined by Law et al (1995:253). They suggested that client-centred practice was:

> an approach to providing occupational therapy which embraces a philosophy of respect for and partnership with people receiving services. It recognises the autonomy of individuals, the need for client choice in making decisions about occupational needs, the strength clients bring to an occupational therapy encounter and the benefits of the client–therapist partnership and the need to ensure that services are accessible and fit the context in which a client lives.

Sumsion (2000:308) conducted research involving therapists throughout the United Kingdom to create the following definition that builds on some of the concepts outlined by Law et al (1995):

> Client-centered occupational therapy is a partnership between the client and the therapist that empowers the client to engage in functional performance and fulfill his or her occupational roles in a variety of environments. The client participates actively in negotiating goals which are given priority and are at the centre of assessment, intervention and evaluation. Throughout the process the therapist listens to and respects the client's values, adapts the interventions to meet the client's needs and enables the client to make informed decisions.

The Canadian Association of Occupational Therapists has been instrumental in moving our thinking forward regarding a client-centred approach. Their definition supports some earlier concepts and adds new issues for consideration. That definition is as follows:

> Client-centered practice refers to collaborative approaches aimed at enabling occupation with clients who may be individuals, groups, agencies, governments, corporations or others. Occupational therapists demonstrate respect for clients, involve clients in decision making, advocate with and for clients in meeting clients' needs, and otherwise recognize clients' experience and knowledge.
>
> (CAOT, 2002:49)

In addition, this professional association has also outlined a relevant model that contains components for therapists to consider if they choose to apply this approach. The Canadian Model of Occupational Performance (CMOP) (CAOT, 2002) reminds practitioners that all aspects of the individual must be considered, including their spirituality, affective, cognitive and physical functioning and challenges, and their self-care, productivity and leisure challenges and goals. All of this occurs within a range of environments that must also be considered and discussed, including the physical, cultural, social and institutional. This model and most of the definitions that have been provided originate in occupational therapy literature. However, the issues they raise including communication, respect, active participation in goal setting, advocacy and choice are relevant to all professionals regardless of the focus of your intervention.

From a clinical perspective the application of any of the components provided in these definitions means that the therapist must clearly outline for the client how they apply a client-centred approach within a specific working environment, and then show by example how the components, including clear communication and respect, will be applied. The essential component underlying any definition you choose is the assurance that the clients' voice is heard and that they are treated with respect (Bibyk et al, 1999; Landers & McCarthy, 2007). From a client-centred perspective the one-size-fits-all approach is not appropriate and therapists are challenged to ensure they are addressing the issues that are of importance to the client (Zandbelt et al, 2006).

Implementation challenges and suggestions for success

A great deal has already been written about the components of client-centred practice and the challenges to be considered when contemplating the use of this approach. The reader is referred to the texts listed at the end of the chapter for more detailed consideration of these issues. This chapter will focus on three of the major implementation challenges – communication, resources and context – as well as some discussion about the client's diagnosis, and the issues of age, gender and attitude.

Communication

Communication is one of the key challenges when implementing a client-centred approach as it becomes extremely important from the first point of contact with the client. Iezzoni (2006) concluded in her literature review that clinical outcomes are actually enhanced by good communication. Each client that walks through the door presents a new scenario and therefore the approach used has to be unique for each individual. Please note that in this chapter the client is considered to be an individual but all of the challenges are only multiplied when the client becomes a group or organisation.

In the first meeting with the client it is very important for therapists to outline what they mean when stating that they work in a client-centred way, as many clients have never heard of this phrase (Maitra & Erway, 2006). An example might be as follows:

> Mrs. Wilson, my name is Dorothy and I am the occupational therapist who will be working with you to address some of the problems you are facing. I need to let you know that I work in a client-centred way which means that you will be fully involved in all of the decisions we make about the problems we will address and how we will work on them. So to begin, can you please tell me about the things that you are having difficulty doing at home?

One of the first important aspects of communication is listening. In fact, Masterson (2007) places listening to find out what is most important to the client as the main defining principle in client-centred practice. However, as healthcare practitioners we are guilty of not listening (Iezzoni, 2006). Nordehn et al (2006) found that all of the participants in their study wanted to be listened to. This involves taking the time to clearly understand the uniqueness of the situation each person faces and not reaching conclusions quickly, based on either what you think the client is saying or trying to say, or previous experience you have had in similar situations. It is important to identify the client's ideas and all of the associated issues such as emotions that relate to their problems (Stewart et al, 2003). You really need to understand their view of their problem and suggestions for dealing with it (Zandbelt et al, 2006). A relevant example here relates to an elderly man involved in an intensive rehabilitation programme following spinal surgery. The team in the rehabilitation centre did not listen to him when he told them he would drive his car again and also walk up the stairs to the second level of his century home. They proceeded to design a programme and follow-up care that involved him remaining in a wheelchair. I am pleased to report that he did meet his goals but sad to reflect on how much more fulfilling his rehabilitation programme would have been if the team had listened to him.

The process then proceeds to the determination of shared goals, expectations and boundaries. To date two studies within occupational therapy have determined that one of the main obstacles to the successful implementation of client-centred practice is that the therapist and clients do not share common goals (Townsend, 1999; Sumsion and Smyth, 2000; Wressle and Samuelsson, 2004). Others have also found that clinicians neglected to share decision making with the clients and, even though they were able to discuss broad concepts such as sharing power, they did not always apply this to their practice (Gillespie et al, 2004). Early discussion of differing views will clarify suggested actions and assist both parties in being true to what they value (Restall et al, 2003). These concerns have been addressed elsewhere (Sumsion, 2007) but I truly believe one of the best ways to implement this approach is to try and apply it to yourself. Successful application of client-centred practice requires the skill of reflection and here is one of the best places to exemplify that skill. Reflect on your reaction to someone you meet for the first time who clearly has a preset agenda and is not the least bit interested in really getting to know you as an individual. How do you react? Personally I shut down and look for the first opportunity to exit from the situation. If that is how your client feels then you have already failed at your attempt to be a client-centred therapist.

Another important aspect of communication is showing respect. We do this by listening carefully, being open to the information the client is trying to convey to us and being willing to learn from the client (Nordehn et al, 2006). Clients have also expressed that respect involves provision of basic information, valuing their intelligence and desire to be informed and to participate in their healthcare (Iezzoni, 2006). Communication also involves conveying the information that the client needs to make decisions and explaining this information thoroughly so the client clearly understands what you are saying (Sumsion, 2005; Nordehn et al, 2006). This information may need to be adjusted according to the client's level of interest, ability to absorb the information and their prior knowledge of both the condition they are facing and therapy services (Lowes, 1998). There are many ways to convey information, including verbally, distribution of written pamphlets and fact sheets. Obviously communication will also need to be adjusted for those with communication challenges, such as some clients in nursing homes (Skinder-Meredith et al, 2007) or with those who have been declared incompetent (Moats, 2007). Another important issue is not to use technical language or assume the client understands what you are saying (Redfern et al, 2006). Spend some time with the client to determine what method works best for them and give them time to absorb what you are saying as well as time to ensure all of their questions are answered.

Overall, from a client-centred perspective, clients continue to report dissatisfaction with communication (Iezzoni, 2006). However, its importance has been shown in women with cancer who had more long-term success with their medication if they were involved in decisions and received relevant information (Kahn et al, 2007). Communication needs to be open and honest as this will help to ensure that clients are fully engaged in the rehabilitation process (Maitra & Erway, 2006).

Resources

As humans we appear to be prone to looking for reasons why something will not work rather than the opposite approach. I am not a psychology expert so I have no idea why this occurs but surely if our main focus is on the clients, then it is our responsibility to take a positive approach. There is always going to be a lack of resources of all types but we cannot let this preclude us from being client-centred (Landers & McCarthy, 2007).

Time is the resource that gets the most attention from a client-centred perspective as we must all simply acknowledge that there will never be enough of it and therapists are short of time (Sumsion & Smyth, 2000; Wilkins et al, 2001). There is a fear that using this approach will consume more time. However, many authors have written with ideas of how to overcome this fear. For example, Lowes (1998) suggests that rephrasing questions to elicit the information you want from the client rather than interrupting them all the time will not increase the time required in the initial visits. It does take more time to ensure clients and their families have the information they need (West et al, 2005).

However, clients have stated that they want and need practitioners to take the time to listen and talk things through with them (Corring and Cook, 1999). The amount of time needed for each client will vary depending on the severity of the issues to be addressed (Sumsion, 2004). However, a basic concept of client-centred practice is that we do take the time to understand the person's story or we will not be able to work in partnership with them to meet their goals.

There are also other resource issues to consider, including type of facility, space and training. Some types of facilities, such as long-term care versus short-term, may be more conducive to applying a client-centred approach. There may also be facilities that choose not to focus on the client's goals which makes application quite a challenge (Maitra & Erway, 2006). Within the facility there may also be differing views between managers and front-line workers as to the resources that are actually required to implement this approach. These differing views may focus the resources on systems and organisations rather than on the client (Gillespie et al, 2004). The available space and design of the facility may also make it challenging to convey information to clients and families in a confidential manner (West et al, 2005).

Hopefully it is becoming clear that client-centred practice is not for the faint of heart as you might have to tackle the system to obtain the resources needed to achieve the clients' goals. It is also important to acknowledge that sometimes success is elusive but that is also part of the reality of life. I recall working with a group of adolescents that were very difficult to motivate. Ultimately they decided they wanted to do a car wash which I embraced with enthusiasm. Their part of this partnership was to prepare the posters and make a list of the supplies they would need. My part was to get the permission of the facility to use their water source. They succeeded and I failed as the facility was not prepared to entertain the liability issues that might arise if a car was damaged. From a client-centred perspective this led to an in-depth discussion of the lessons we had all learned and how we could apply this to challenges they would face in the community. We did not fail. We learned.

The application of a client-centred approach is not an automatic process. It takes knowledge, training and practice to be able to use this approach effectively. In one study the application barrier ranked the highest by occupational therapists was not having enough knowledge about this approach (Wressle & Samuelsson, 2004). The nurses in a study conducted by West et al (2005) clearly stated that they would welcome more training, especially in areas that the clients identified had failed to meet their expectations.

Context

Context includes the variety of healthcare environments in which therapists work that were mentioned above (Restall et al, 2003). Within these contexts it is important that management and front-line staff work together with clients, including families, to implement change effectively (Wilkins et al, 2001). However, the concept is broader than those issues. Reference to the Canadian Model of Occupational Performance (CAOT, 2002) will clearly show the reader that the context of the intervention is a very important consideration in client-centred practice. Within the model the context relates to the social, cultural, institutional (including political, legal and economic considerations) and physical environments with which the client engages. Some of these environments are more complex than others. For example Iwama (1999) reminds us that within the Japanese culture this approach must include traditional values and beliefs. This context can either enhance or limit that application of this approach (Landers & McCarthy, 2007). This context must also include and consider others in the environment that will be impacted by goals chosen and decisions made (Dalley, 1999). Returning a client with a new found enthusiasm for education to a community that does not support this goal, or a client to an independent living situation when the family feels this is a big mistake may not lead to the attainment of the client's goals.

Diagnoses

The people with whom one works from a client-centred perspective are experiencing a problem of some kind and probably a fairly significant illness or diagnosis. Think about how you feel when you are ill and how that interferes with your normal function. In this state you are less likely to readily make decisions and determine exactly what the priorities are. Due to their diagnoses clients may have decreased cognition, be unable to verbalise their concerns or be unmotivated (Maitra & Erway, 2006). Sumsion (2005) also found that the severity of the client's illness posed major challenges. One client in this study stated clearly that even with all the assistance available she just simply might reach a point where she could not take advantage of what was on offer to her.

Age and gender

Hopefully it is clear by this point in the chapter that applying a client-centred approach requires the practitioner to engage in a considerable amount of reflection. There is no cookbook for this approach that will tell you exactly what to do in all situations. The best way to handle most interactions is to use yourself as a barometer and ask how you would feel and/or react if you were in the client's position. This is especially true when we consider the question of age and gender. As young people entering your profession how do you react when older people tell you how something should be done? Reverse that thinking and consider how an older client will react to you as a younger person who has more expertise with the problems they are facing. Maitra and Erway (2006) found that younger clients participated more in goal setting than did older clients. On reflection one can hopefully realise that this makes perfect sense. Older clients come from an era when you simply did what you were told by the medical profession, so asking them what their goals are may be a foreign concept. The therapists in Sumsion's study (2004) also identified that the older clients just wanted the therapist to tell them what to do.

The second issue to consider here is that of gender. There is no need for this to be a major challenge but it does need to be considered. Again the therapists Sumsion (2004) interviewed felt that gender did have an impact on their ability to apply a client-centred approach. They expressed that clients were more accepting of a female therapist and that the male clients found it easier to talk to them. However, they also realised that older men found it difficult to express some issues to a younger female, and the male therapists had a number of things to consider if the potential existed to be alone with a female client.

Attitude

Is it possible that the attitudes of therapists are preventing the effective application of client-centred practice? This approach does require a willingness to redistribute power which some therapists may be unwilling to do (Gillespie et al, 2004). The clients in one study very clearly identified that therapists had negative attitudes and used words such as derogatory and sarcastic to describe their reactions to the staff (Corring & Cook, 1999).

Summary

This chapter aimed to assist the reader with the identification of key challenges when attempting to implement client-centred practice, as well as to suggest some strategies that could be implemented to address these challenges. Issues, arising from relevant definitions, were identified that need to be addressed before successful implementation can occur. These issues included communication, acknowledgment of resources and related limitations, clarification of context, issues related to the client's diagnosis, age and gender of both the client and the therapist and therapists' attitudes. There is no cookbook or specific recipe or direction for addressing each of these issues successfully. That success comes only from the therapist's knowledge base and willingness to be a reflective practitioner, who considers each issue in relation to oneself and as a result comes to know oneself much better (Masterson,

2007). Client-centred practice has been a significant component of occupational therapy since the early 1980s and the issues outlined in this chapter have been active since that time. Surely this tells us that the system is incapable of addressing them, but each therapist can address them successfully within the client partnership. Overall, the uniqueness of the client-centred approach comes from approaching each client as a unique and separate entity and by striving to understand their story, beliefs, concerns and boundaries (Schoot et al, 2005). I personally believe that all clients deserve the benefits that arise from this approach and hope and trust that you will do your utmost to ensure they benefit from a client-centred approach.

Further reading

Canadian Association of Occupational Therapists (2002) *Enabling Occupation: an Occupational Therapy Perspective*. Ottawa: CAOT Publications ACE.

Gertais, M., Edgman-Levitan, S., Daley, J., Delbanco, T.L. (eds) (1993) *Through the Patient's Eyes: Understanding and Promoting Patient-Centered Care*. San Francisco: Jossey-Bass Publishers.

Law, M. (ed) (1998) *Client-Centered Occupational Therapy*. New Jersey: Slack Incorporated.

Stewart, M., Belle Brown, J., Weston, W.W., McWhinney, I.R., McWilliam, C., Freeman, T.R. (2003) *Patient-Centred Medicine: Transforming the Clinical Method*, 2nd edn. Oxford: Radcliffe Medical Press Ltd.

Sumsion, T. (ed) (2006) *Client-centred Practice in Occupational Therapy: A Guide to Implementation*, 2nd edn. Edinburgh: Churchill Livingstone.

Townsend, E.A., Polatajko, H.J. (2007) *Enabling Occupation 11: Advancing an Occupational Therapy Vision for Health, Wellbeing & Justice Through Occupation*. Ottawa: CAOT Publications ACE.

References

Bibyk, B., Day, D.G., Morris, M. et al. (1999) Who's in charge here? The client's perspective on client-centred care. *OT Now*, September/October, 11–12.

Brown, T.A. (2001) Five ways to run a successful patient-centred practice. *Ontario Dentist* May, 10–11.

Canadian Association of Occupational Therapists (2002) *Enabling Occupation: an Occupational Therapy Perspective*, 2nd edn. Ottawa: CAOT Publications ACE.

College of Occupational Therapists (2005) *Code of Ethics and Professional Conduct*. Available online: http://www.cot.org.uk

Corring, D., Cook, J. (1999) Client-centred care means that I am a valued human being. *Canadian Journal of Occupational Therapy* **66**(2), 71–82.

Dalley, J. (1999) Evaluation of clinical practice. *Physiotherapy* **85**(9), 491–497.

Epstein, R.M. (2000) The science of patient-centered care. *The Journal of Family Practice* **49**(9), 805–807.

Gillespie, R., Florin, D., Gillam, S. (2004) How is patient-centred care understood by the clinical, managerial and lay stakeholders responsible for promoting this agenda? *Health Expectations* **7**(2), 142–148.

Iezzoni, L.I. (2006) Make no assumptions: communication between persons with disabilities and clinicians. *Assistive Technology* **18**(2), 212–219.

Iwama, M. (1999) Cross-cultural perspectives on client-centred occupational therapy practice: a view from Japan. *OT Now* **1**, 4–6

Kahn, K.L., Schneider, E.C., Malin, J.L., Adams, J.L., Epstein, A.M. (2007) Patient centered experiences in breast cancer: predicting long-term adherence to tamoxifen use. *Medical Care* **45**(5), 431–439.

Landers, M.G., McCarthy, G.M. (2007) Person-centered nursing practice with older people in Ireland. *Nursing Science Quarterly* **20**(1), 78–84.

Law, M., Baptiste, S., Mills, J. (1995) Client centred practice: what does it mean and does it make a difference? *Canadian Journal of Occupational Therapy* **62**(5), 250–257.

Lowes, R. (1998) Patient-centered care for better patient adherence. *Family Practice Management* **5**(3), 46–47, 51–54, 57.

Maitra, K.K., Erway, F. (2006) Perception of client-centered practice in occupational therapists and their clients. *The American Journal of Occupational Therapy* **60**(3), 298–310.

Masterson, A. (2007) Community matrons: person-centred care planning (part one). *Nursing Older People* **19**(4), 23–26.

Moats, M. (2007) Discharge decision-making, enabling occupations and client-centred practice. *Canadian Journal of Occupational Therapy* **74**(2), 91–101.

Nordehn, G., Meredith, A., Bye, L. (2006) A preliminary investigation of barriers to achieving patient-centered communication with patients who have stroke-related communication disorders. *Topics in Stroke Rehabilitation* **13**(1), 68–77.

Redfern, J., Mckevitt, C., Wolfe, C.D.A. (2006) Risk management after stroke: the limits of a patient-centred approach. *Health, Risk & Society* **8**(2), 123–141.

Restall, G., Ripat, J., Stern, M. (2003) A framework of strategies for client-centred practice. *Canadian Journal of Occupational Therapy* **70**(2),103–112.

Schoot, T., Proot, I., ter Meulen, R., deWitte, L. (2005) Recognition of client values as a basis for tailored care: the view of Dutch expert patients and family caregivers. *Scandinavian Journal of Caring Sciences* **19**(2), 169–176.

Skinder-Meredith, A., Bye, L., Bulthuis, K., Schueller, A. (2007) Patient-centered communication survey of nursing homes and rehabilitation centers. *The Journal of Long Term Home Health Care* **8**(1), 8–15.

Stewart, M., Belle Brown, J., Weston, W.W., McWhinney, I.R., McWilliam, C., Freeman, T.R. (2003) *Patient-centred medicine: Transforming the clinical method*, 2nd edn. Oxford: Radcliffe Medical Press Ltd.

Sumsion, T. (2000) A revised occupational therapy definition of client-centred practice. *British Journal of Occupational Therapy* **63**(7), 304–309.

Sumsion, T. (2004) Pursuing the client's goals really paid off. *British Journal of Occupational Therapy* **67**, 2–9.

Sumsion, T. (2005) Facilitating client-centred practice: Insights from clients. *Canadian Journal of Occupational Therapy* **72**(1), 13–20.

Sumsion, T. (2007) The art of person and community centred practice. Submitted for inclusion in: M. Curtin, M. Molineux and J. Supyk (eds) *Turners Occupational Therapy and Physical Dysfunction*, 6th edn. Oxford: Elsevier.

Sumsion, T., Smyth, G. (2000) Barriers to client-centredness and their resolution. *Canadian Journal of Occupational Therapy*, **67**(1), 15–21.

Townsend, L. (1999) Client-centred practice: good intentions overruled. *OT Now* **1**:14–15.

West, E., Barron, D.N., Reeves, R. (2005) Overcoming the barriers to patient-centred care: time, tools and training. *Journal of Clinical Nursing* **14**, 435–443.

Wilkins, S., Pollock, N., Rochon, S., Law, M. (2001) Implementing client-centred practice: why is it so difficult to do? *Canadian Journal of Occupational Therapy* **68**(2), 70–79.

Wressle, E., Samuelsson, K. (2004) Barriers and bridges to client-centred occupational therapy in Sweden. *Scandinavian Journal of Occupational Therapy* **11**(1), 12–16.

Zandbelt, L.C., Smets, E.M.A., Oort, F.J., Godfried, M.H., deHaes, H.C.J.M. (2006) Determinants of physicians' patient-centred behaviour in the medical specialist encounter. *Social Science & Medicine* **63**(4), 899–910.

5: Empowerment in the context of practice: The times they are a-changin'

Margaret Gallagher and Elizabeth Cassidy

Why do we need to understand service user empowerment today, when we are all expected to be client- or patient-centred in our practice? As with other fundamental principles of practice, being a therapist who empowers the service user requires personal insight and a sophisticated approach to practice. This chapter explains the background, relevance and principles of service user empowerment in contemporary healthcare and social practice. Empowerment is a challenging element in the dialogue between health and social care professionals and service users. We argue that effective empowerment requires a shift in current practice. This is important for healthcare professionals as there is evidence that empowering patients leads to their increasing independence (Langer & Rodin, 1976) and care that dis-empowers patients increases their dependence (Conwill, 1993).

The term empowerment sits within an abundant lexicon, including client-centred practice, choice, participation, enablement, partnership, collaboration and user-led services. Acknowledging the importance of these terms, we don't seek to define them in the context of empowerment but to explore the implications of practising as an empowering therapist. For the purposes of this chapter we will use the term service user to include patients, clients and carers.

Definitions of empowerment

Internationally, the concept of patient empowerment came from the health improvement movement in the 1970s (Lewin, 2006), and is described by Tones (1998:71) as 'complex and slippery'; it relates to the reciprocal relationship between the individual and their environment. This complexity may explain the lack of articulation in government policy. In the UK the idea of empowerment emerged from the community activism of the 1960s and 1970s (Gibson, 1991) and is an umbrella term, sheltering many concepts (Elliott and Turrell, 1996).

Gibson's definition in relation to nursing provided clarity about the concept in healthcare:

> a social process of recognising, promoting and enhancing people's abilities to meet their own needs, solve their own problems and mobilise the necessary resources in order to feel in control of their own lives.
>
> (Gibson, 1991:359)

Whilst recognising the individual level highlighted by Zimmerman (1990), Gilbert (1991) sets a much broader context for describing the context of empowerment, developing it from an individual process to one set within a societal context and including organisational and community perspectives.

Lewin (2006), when reviewing the empowerment literature, identifies four dimensions of empowerment, which may be a more useful perspective for therapists to consider for incorporating into clinical practice. These are:

- the individual patient's beliefs and abilities to have power, influence and control;
- the willingness and commitment of healthcare professionals to empower patients;
- a perceived change in the power or control over their care by patients;
- equality of opportunity and freedom from discrimination.

These four dimensions examine the implicit power relationships inherent in clinical practice as well as recognising the oppressive behaviours within society.

Therefore the central elements within empowerment are: the redistribution of power between patients and professionals; removing power from service providers; and facilitating 'a patient's sense of control over their well being' (Nyatanga, 2002:235), including their growth and development (Kuokkanen, 2000).

Townsend and Polatajko (2007) suggest that therapists should share power with their clients in order for them to make decisions. There is evidence from nursing that the authority vested in such professionals acts as a barrier to patient empowerment (Nyatanga, 2002). This appears to indicate that the traditional professional hierarchies also have a role in sustaining the imbalance of power between service users and professionals.

International perspective

The Ottawa Charter (1986), from the World Health Organization's (WHO) first conference on health promotion, focused on the empowerment of individuals and communities. This informed the WHO framework for measuring health and disability, the International Classification of Functioning Disability and Health (ICF) (WHO, 2001), which places all health conditions within broad socio-political contexts (see Chapter 8). The role of the health professional to advocate, enable and mediate on behalf of individuals is central to the framework, and has been aligned with the Canadian Model of Occupational Engagement (Townsend & Polatajko, 2007).

For occupational therapists, empowerment is defined as working 'with clients, in reaching towards visions of possibility for occupational dreams and futures' (Townsend & Polatajko 2007:92) and it is subsumed in key concepts, such as client-centred practice (see Chapter 4) as a component of the approach to practice (Wilcock, 2006).

Context: the view from the United Kingdom

The need for greater transparency and accountability to the public has been fostered by a number of service failures, such as the Bristol Royal Infirmary Inquiry (2001) and the Shipman Inquiry (2001). From these inquiries, a drive emerged to improve the public accountability of health and social services with recommendations to include the public and service users in the design and delivery of services (Calnan & Gabe, 2001). The Health Professions Council enshrines such notions of public accountability and transparency in the Standards of Practice Conduct, Performance and Ethics (HPC, 2004). Two important components of empowerment are the provision of information and an effective complaints procedure, but we would argue that this gives a narrow interpretation of empowerment.

Gibson (1991) suggests that, for empowerment to work, there has to be a critical shift in practice through which healthcare professionals relinquish power and share it with the service user, requiring health professionals to facilitate this process. Sanderson (1999) suggests that 'institutional changes are not enough to promote empowerment'. There are concerns about the mismatch between the use of the medical model and the adoption of the concept of empowerment (Wilcock, 2006). The power relationships engendered by the medical model in acute care do not support the sharing of power. Moving from what Anderson and Funnell (2004) term the acute-care paradigm, with which we are all familiar, will require a shift in practice.

> Empowerment approach would aim to involve users in the development, management and operation of services as well as in the assessment of need.
>
> (Barnes & Walker, 1998:379)

In such a sharing of responsibility and authority lies the opportunity to support self-efficacy for service users and collaborative partnerships between service stakeholders.

The Commission for Patient and Public Involvement in Health (2007) continues the policy drive to empower communities by making services more accountable.

Service users' understanding of the societal context of service design and delivery, including awareness that they may experience discrimination, is a vital part of their empowerment (Means et al, 2003). How the service users are informed and supported to make appropriate choices is a concern outlined by the Sainsbury Centre for Mental Health (2006). The Expert Patients programme has aimed to empower patients with knowledge and responsibility for their conditions, and facilitate their contribution to service design and delivery (Department of Health, 2001). Current government policy attempts to address social inclusion for historically marginalised groups, such as women, children and ethnic minorities, involving the public in decisions that affect people's health and well-being (Commission for Patient and Public Involvement in Health, 2007). Professional bodies, such as the College of Occupational Therapists, have integrated the user-led service perspective into policy guidance (COT, 2006). The Chartered Society of Physiotherapists has embedded the principles of empowerment in the Rules of Professional Conduct (CSP, 2005).

Empowerment in practice

User empowerment is the highest level of patient and carer participation in healthcare, signifying a shift in power towards individuals, groups, organisations and communities from what is traditionally a professionally dominated environment (Poulton, 1999). The extent to which patients feel empowered and in control as individuals is likely to depend at least in part on their interactions with healthcare practitioners (Jones et al, 2000). Therapists, therefore, need to develop skills and strategies to work with patients as partners. Therapists who work in successful partnership with their patients are those who respect their patients' expertise and experience as a valuable resource (Edwards et al, 2004; Wikman & Faltholm, 2006). Therefore empowerment in practice means engaging patients and carers in collaborative working and addressing practices, behaviours and assumptions that engender and perpetuate helplessness and alienation. The experience of collaboration and power sharing may be transformative for both the therapist and the patient or carer through the production of new knowledge and perspectives that may challenge pre-existing assumptions (Edwards et al, 2004). It is therefore crucial that practitioners develop skill in critical self-reflection to improve practice and to support patients and carers to gain control on their own terms (Jones et al, 2000).

Relinquishing control and power does not necessarily come naturally to healthcare practitioners. Thornquist (2001:159) conducted a qualitative study of physiotherapists' first encounter with patients and described the difficulty that some physiotherapists had in letting go of their expert status; 'therapists do what they know best because it makes them feel that they are master of the situation'. This attitude was found with particular reference to psychosocial and contextual issues, where little weight was given to patients' concerns and experiences. Wottrich et al (2004) looked at the characteristics of physiotherapy from the patients' and therapists' perspective. Major differences were revealed. For example, the importance physiotherapists claimed they attached to empowering patients was not confirmed with patients and the extent to which the physiotherapists believed they considered the patient's previous experience and knowledge during treatment sessions was also contested.

Kerssens et al (1999) explored the content of back care information provided by physiotherapists. The authors found that back care information was not tailored to individual patient's needs or contexts and that the number of instructions in the back care programmes was determined by the therapist rather than the patient. The authors recommended that individualised instructions tailored to the patient's specific needs and circumstances would, in this case, improve patient 'adherence' (Kerssens et al, 1999:294). Further evidence suggests that a less autocratic approach to exercise prescription, through giving patients control over exercise and feedback conditions, not only benefits the therapeutic relationship in terms of empowerment but actively enhances learning in certain rehabilitation situations (McNevin et al, 2000).

Healthcare practitioners need to recognise and be mindful of the difficulties they may have in relinquishing power and how this may influence patients' experiences. It would seem that, as junior or novice practitioners may not have the same degree of skill as their more experienced colleagues, they are more likely to fall back on a prescriptive model of intervention where opportunity for collaboration and empowerment is minimal. Benner (1984) proposed that as practitioners become more expert they are able to challenge preconceived ideas and appreciate the subtleties that individual patients bring to practice situations. Expertise involves skills in interpretation of information and the application of 'discretionary judgement' that often transcends standard rules and guidelines for practice (Benner, 1984:177). However, expertise is situational; faced with new or more complex challenges, experienced practitioners may perform at a lower level of expertise and be less able to understand and respond to the needs of individual patients (Benner, 1984). More recently Thornquist (2001) suggested that experienced practitioners are also at risk of using habituated practice rather than individualised practice, even when the comfortable and familiar is not the most appropriate course of action. Critical self-reflection and mentoring should be used by both novice and experienced practitioners to develop practices that enhance rather than stifle collaboration and empowerment, particularly in new or complex situations.

Empowerment through mutual enquiry

Jensen et al (2002:332) developed an approach to physiotherapy termed the patient–practitioner collaborative model. Although designed with physiotherapy in mind it could apply equally to other healthcare practice. The model consists of four stages: establishing the therapeutic relationship; diagnosing through mutual enquiry; finding common ground through negotiation; and intervention and follow-up.

Barr and Threlkeld (2000) used an earlier version of the collaborative model to describe the process of developing a treatment plan to treat a patient's physical limitations whilst addressing both personal and social domains. Critical steps in the successful treatment of this patient were identified by the authors. For example the patient was resistant to using any form of walking aid due to a perceived loss of independence; he also had difficulty accepting that his gait pattern had any influence on his low back pain. This potential 'deal breaker' was identified through mutual enquiry and resolved through information sharing, discussion of assessment findings and negotiation. The patient refused crutches but agreed to use a collapsible stick to reduce adverse biomechanical influences on his low back pain. Without a relinquishing of power by the therapist it is unlikely that the outcome of treatment would have been as successful.

Even when the opportunities for mutual enquiry seem slim it is still possible to work from an empowering perspective. Tannous et al (1999) interviewed experienced occupational therapists about their views on working with clients with learning disability. Priority outcomes for clients were regarded as achieving autonomy, self-determination and community integration. There were several instances where occupational therapists seemed to be working from an empowering perspective. There were examples of direct empowerment (enabling a child to choose and therefore control when she wanted food to be brought to her mouth), as well as indirect empowerment (an occupational therapist was able to change the attitudes and perceptions of others through their observation of her work with a child with learning difficulties).

The lessons that may be drawn from these examples are that working from an empowering perspective is possible, even in challenging situations, and that power shifts are possible when the therapist challenges their own assumptions and works collaboratively with patients and carers. There is a need for further research to demonstrate the effect of service user empowerment on practice, as the above examples illustrate how this can affect our practice.

The service user's voice

Partnerships with voluntary organisations provide opportunities to develop services that are empowering from the perspective of the service user. The voluntary sector provides guidance for the development of user-led services, emphasising the user-led organization model for services for disabled people 'Making user involvement work' (Joseph Rowntree Foundation, 2006). The voluntary sector's role in this is currently focused through the National Voices initiative (2007). User involvement and empowerment can realign the relationships between service users and healthcare professionals to influence individual's health status, and change the culture of healthcare (Tritter & McCrum, 2005).

However, initiatives to involve the public and service users may not empower them (Calnan & Gabe, 2001). It is interesting to note that from a doctor's perspective, patients are reminded of their responsibilities as well as their rights (Taylor, 2000), possibly hinting that there is some resistance to the rebalancing of the power relationship between doctors and their patients. There is also evidence that practitioners, such as nurses, are not prepared to share their power with patients (Henderson, 2003). A study of empowerment in a coronary care unit demonstrated that patients are content to leave decisions to professionals (Lewin, 2006). Calnan and Gabe (2001) are sceptical regarding either patients' ability to take responsibility for decision making, or that doctors have the appropriate skills to share the decision-making process. The above tensions and the question about who is driving or benefiting from the empowerment debate is a question for further research and personal consideration (Lewin, 2006).

Acknowledging the complexity and potential for negative compromise, we suggest that the service users' voice, both individually and collectively, needs to be integral to all aspects of service development and delivery. The indications are that taking a partnership approach with service users would provide more appropriate services for them.

Making it happen

Integrating service user empowerment into practice requires a significant shift in health professionals' approach to their practice (Gibson, 2001). Moving from the paternalistic, medical model of practice to a client-centred social model of intervention will need a whole system approach to include the public, health and social care professionals, service providers and the voluntary sectors all taking responsibility for embedding this in practice. Education and support of service users are also central to making this an enduring approach to delivering health and social care in the twenty-first century. The hope is that the negative history of tokenistic inclusion of the public and service users will positively inform the shape of current and future service development. Health professionals need to be mindful that, for service user empowerment to succeed, financial resources are required and there needs to be commitment from health and social care professionals (Sainsbury Centre for Mental Health, 2006).

We suggest that the following approaches will support the development of an empowering approach in practice.

Reflective practice

Using reflection to gain insight into our individual processes is an important aspect of empowering practice behaviours and in the development of clinical reasoning skills. This is discussed in more depth in Chapter 3.

Recovery model

Mental health services promote the recovery model, where hope, autonomy, self-determination and service user participation are key elements of the approach (Oades et al, 2005). The service user owns the process, defining goals, including employment, education and training as part of the recovery process, promoting collaboration between service users and professionals as described by Masterson (2006:31):

> The empowerment of individuals must include the fostering of positive, client-centred relationships for the psychological empowerment, as well as the formal transfer of powers of decision-making for consumerist empowerment.

The recovery model demonstrates commitment to client-centred practice, which healthcare professionals understand to be a core element of practice. Currently practice in healthcare is frequently delivered through the medical model but, for empowerment to work effectively for service users and the practitioners, the recovery model provides a way of developing a partnership approach. The use of the recovery model may assist the complex conversations within interdisciplinary working, in order to shift practice and provide a service which is truly client centred.

Evaluation

An important part of establishing if service user empowerment is working is to evaluate the approach adopted. One model used in hospital environments, the Patient Empowerment Scale, considers nurse/patient

Box 5.1 A vehicle of hope

This is the view of a junior therapist working in a mental health setting where the recovery model is used:

> Working with the recovery model has never made me feel like I am relinquishing power, it always feels like I am adding more fuel to this vehicle of hope or something like that and it can create quite a dynamic relationship between me and the client.

interaction (Faulkner, 2001). It is described as a patient empowerment awareness tool to analyse the interactions between nursing staff and patients. Given the limited research in this area, audit and evaluation are a good place to start in terms both of research and of providing guidance for good practice.

Summary of key points

Will empowerment herald a new way of working with our service users? Times may be a-changin', but the pace maybe too slow for some stakeholders who want to see more radical evidence of progress to a user-led service. It is likely that, to achieve this shift in practice, it will take a generation, and will require finance and commitment from all those involved in the health and social care arena including service users, professional bodies, the statutory agencies and education.

The fundamental redistribution of power within the relationships health and social care professionals have with service users will require new ways of thinking about our practice. Reflective practice, mutual inquiry, models of practice such as the recovery models, plus practice evaluation and research to establish best practice, offer opportunities to support the empowerment of service users. Partnerships with the voluntary sector can prove to be a powerful agent for change in practising as an empowering therapist. The concept and practice of service user empowerment remains an aim for all health and social care professionals. However only time will tell whether service user empowerment is embedded in practice, or just the most recent fad that will fade from both policy directives and practice aspirations.

Exercise to evaluate learning

Read the two case studies (Boxes 5.2 and 5.3) and then answer the questions below.

Box 5.2 Case one

A patient on an acute respiratory care ward was recovering from surgery when another patient was admitted to the ward in a distressed state. A nurse spent time speaking to the new patient in the hope that she would become calmer. However this patient remained anxious and the nurse asked the recovering patient to speak to the new patient about her time on the ward. This conversation had very positive results, as the new patient settled and the recovering patient felt trusted by the nurse, apparently gaining authority from the nurse. The empowerment of the recovering patient made her feel valued by the nurse, and this supported a relationship of trust between them.

> **Box 5.3** Case two
>
> I am currently working with a client with a long history of mental health problems who is determined to return to work. In the past few weeks I have referred and accompanied her to a local employment service that specialises in placing people in appropriate voluntary or paid positions.
>
> My client's journey back to employment has been hampered by her low mood and poor organisational skills. I have often made appointments for her at employment that she cancelled at the last minute. More recently when she asked me to cancel her appointment I urged her to cancel the appointment herself and rearrange a time that was more suitable for her. She appeared very anxious at the thought of having to do this but nevertheless made another appointment for herself.
>
> It has not always been easy for her. She attended an appointment on the wrong day which was a source of distress for her. However, she continues to make her own appointments and has even taken on more responsibility. Only this week she asked for my help in filling out a complex vocational self-assessment form. We arranged a time for this but before the time came she proudly approached me and showed me that she had filled out the form herself.

Questions

What are your key reflections from these case studies?

How does this inform your approach to empowerment in practice?

What reflective process have you used to understand these transactions? See Chapter 3.

Would you have done anything differently?

What else could be done in your practice setting?

Were there any barriers to using an empowering approach?

What has supported you to become an empowering therapist?

References

Anderson, R.M., Funnell, M.M. (2004) Patient empowerment: reflections on the challenge of fostering the adoption of a new paradigm. *Patient Education and Counselling* **57**(2), 153–157.

Barnes, M., Walker, A. (1996) Consumerism versus empowerment: a principled approach to the involvement of older service users. *Policy Politics* **24**(4), 375–393.

Barr, J., Threlkeld, A.J. (2000) Patient-practitioner collaboration in clinical decision making. *Physiotherapy Research International* **5**(4), 254–260.

Benner, P. (1984) *From Novice to Expert: Excellence and Power in Clinical Nursing Practice*. Menlo Park, California: Addison-Wesley Publishing Company.

Bristol Royal Infirmary Inquiry (2001) Public Involvement Through Empowerment, Chapter 28 www.bristol-inquiry.org.uk/ (Accessed 28th October 2007).

Calnan, M., Gabe, J. (2001) From consumerism to partnership? Britain's National Health Service at the turn of the century. *International Journal of Health Services* **31**(1), 119–131.

Chartered Society of Physiotherapy (2005) *Core Standards of Practice*. London: Chartered Society of Physiotherapy.

College of Occupational Therapists (2006) *Recovering Ordinary Lives. The strategy for occupational therapy in mental health services 2007–2017, a vision for the next ten years*. London: College of Occupational Therapists.

Commission for Patient and Public Involvement in Health (2007) *Annual Report 2006/7*. London: The Stationery Office.

Conwill, J. (1993) Understanding and combating helplessness. *Rehabilitation Nursing* **18**(6), 388–394.

Department of Health (2001) *The Expert Patient: A New Approach to Chronic Disease Management*. London: The Stationery Office.

Edwards, I., Jones, M. Higgs, J., Trede, F., Jensen, G. (2004) What is collaborative reasoning? *Advances in Physiotherapy* **6**(2), 70–83.

Elliot, M.A., Turrell, A.R. (1996) Dilemmas for the empowering nurse. *Journal of Nursing Management* **4**(5), 273–279.

Faulkner, M. (2001) A measure of patient empowerment in hospital environments catering for older people. *Journal of Advanced Nursing* **34**(5), 676–686.

Gibson, C. (1991) A concept analysis of empowerment. *Journal of Advanced Nursing* **16**(3), 354–361.

Health Professions Council (2004) *Standards of Conduct, Performance and Ethics*, 034/ HPC/A5 April 2004 (reprinted July 2007).

Henderson, S. (2003) Power in balance between nurses and patients: a potential inhibitor of partnership in care. *Journal of Clinical Nursing* **12**, 501–508.

Jensen, G.M., Lorish, C.D., Shepard, K.F. (2002) Understanding and influencing patient receptivity to change: the patient practitioner collaborative model. In: K.F. Shepherd and G.M. Jansen (eds) *Handbook of Teaching for Physical Therapists*, 2nd edn. Oxford: Butterworth Heinemann.

Jones, F., Mandy, A., Partridge, C. (2000) Who's in control after stroke? Do we disempower our patients? *Physiotherapy Research International* **5**(4), 249–253.

Joseph Rowntree Foundation (2006) *Making User Involvement Work*. Joseph Rowntree Foundation, The Homestead, 40 Water End, York YO30 6WP: www.jrf.org.uk (Accessed 31st October 2007).

Kerssens, J.J., Sluijs, E.M., Verhaak, F.M., Knibbe, H.J.J., Hermans, I.M.J. (1999) Back care instructions in physical therapy: a trend analysis of individualised back care programmes. *Physical Therapy* **79**(3), 286–295.

Kuokkanen, L. (2000) Power and empowerment in nursing: three theoretical approaches. *Journal of Advanced Nursing* **31**(1), 235–241.

Langer, E.J., Rodin, J. (1976) The effects of choice and the enhanced personal responsibility for the aged: a field experiment in institutional setting. *Journal of Personality and Social Psychology* **34**(2), 191–198.

Lewin, D. (2006) Patient empowerment within a coronary care unit: Insights for health professionals drawn from a patient satisfaction survey. *Intensive and Critical Care Nursing* **23**(2), 81–90.

Masterson, S. (2006) Mental health service user's social and individual empowerment: using theories of power to elucidate far-reaching strategies. *Journal of Mental Health* **15**(1), 19–34.

Means, R., Richards, S., Randall, S. (2003) *Community Care Policy and Practice*, 3rd edn. England: Palgrave MacMillan.

McNevin, N.H., Wulf, G., Carlson, C. (2000) Effects of attentional focus, self control and dyad training on motor learning: implications for physical therapy. *Physical Therapy* **80**(4), 373–385.

National Voices www.lmca.org.uk/pages/update_on_the_national_voices_project.html (Accessed 28th October 2007).

Nyatanga, L. (2002) Empowerment in nursing: the role of philosophical and psychological factors. *Nursing Philosophy* **3**(3), 234–239.

Oades, L., Deane, F., Crowe, T., Lambert, G., Kavanagh, D., Lloyd, C. (2005) Collaborative recovery: an integrative model for working with individuals who experience chronic and recurring mental illness. *Australian Psychiatry* **13**(3), 279–284.

Ottawa Charter for Health Promotion (1986) *Health and Welfare Canada*. Ottawa, Canada: Canadian Public Health Association.

Poulton, B.C. (1999) User involvement in identifying health needs and shaping and evaluating services: is it being realised? *Journal of Advanced Nursing* **30**(6), 1289–1296.

Sainsbury Centre for Mental Health (2006) *Choices in Mental Health*. Briefing 31. London, England.

Sanderson, I. (1999) Participation and democratic renewal: from instrumental to communicative rationality. *Policy and Politics* **27**(3), 325–341.

Shipman Inquiry (2001) Fifth Report, Chapter 27, Proposals' for Change, **27**,131–132 www.the-shipman-inquiry.org.uk/home.asp (Accessed 31st October 2007).

Tannous, C., Lehmann-Monck, V., Magoffin, R., Jackson, O., Llewellyn, G. (1999) Beyond good practice: issues in working with people with intellectual disability and high support needs. *Australian Occupational Therapy Journal* **46**(1), 24–35.

Taylor, M. (2000) Patient care (empowerment): a local view. *British Medical Journal* **320**, 1663–1664.

Thornquist, E. (2001) Diagnostics in physiotherapy – processes, patterns and perspectives. Part II. *Advances in Physiotherapy* **3**(4), 151–162.

Tones, K. (1998) Health education and promotion of health: seeking wisely to empower. In: S. Kendall (ed) *Health and Empowerment Research and Practice*. London: Arnold.

Townsend, E.A., Polatajko, H.J. (2007) *Enabling Occupation II: Advancing an Occupational Therapy Vision for Health, Well-being, & Justice Through Occupation*. Ottawa, Canada: Canadian Association of Occupational Therapists.

Tritter, J.Q., McCrum, A. (2005) The snakes and ladders of involvement: Moving beyond Arnstein. *Health Policy* **76**(2), 156–168.

Wilcock, A.A. (2006) *An Occupational Perspective of Health*, 2nd edn. New Jersey: Slack Incorporated.

Wikman, A.M., Faltholm, Y. (2006) Patient empowerment in rehabilitation: 'Somebody told me to get rehabilitated'. *Advances in Physiotherapy* **8**(1), 23–32.

World Health Organization (2001) *International Classification of Functioning, Disability and Health*. Geneva, Switzerland: WHO.

Wottrich, A.W., Stenstrom, C.A., Tham, K., von Koch, L. (2004) Characteristics of physiotherapy sessions from the patient's and therapist's perspective. *Disability and Rehabilitation* **26**(2), 1198–1205.

Zimmerman, M. (1990) Towards a theory of learned hopefulness: a structural model of analysis of participation and empowerment. *Journal of Research in Personality* **24**(1), 71–86.

6: Cultural issues in professional practice

Kee Hean Lim

Culture is a term that is often mentioned but not always clearly understood. Assumptions are often made on what the term 'culture' encompasses and how it may impact upon professional practice in health and social care. The focus of this chapter is firstly to define and examine the different meanings of the term 'culture'; secondly, to examine the contextual reasons for its relevance and importance within the UK and beyond; thirdly, to explore how the concept of 'culture', including how the specific issue of professional culture, may impact upon the practice and service delivery of occupational therapy and physiotherapy; fourthly, to challenge novice and experienced health and social care practitioners and providers to examine and reflect upon their practice and equip them with knowledge and skills in pursuit of delivering culturally sensitive, inclusive, safe and effective care.

Although the focus of this chapter is primarily aimed at occupational therapists and physiotherapists, the concepts, issues, challenges and potential solutions indicated are of equal relevance and importance to the wider spectrum of health and social care professions, like nursing, social work, psychology and medicine. As such, the author will draw upon literature across these respective professional disciplines to support the concepts and issues raised within the chapter. Additionally, the terms client and patient will be used interchangeably within the text, further highlighting the differing values placed upon the relationship between the professional groups and the care recipient.

Definitions of key terms

Within this chapter, a definition of key terms is given to reduce the confusion and apprehension that is often associated with discussions around issues of culture. Culture within its most narrow definition may be associated with ethnicity, race and minority ethnic groups (Lim & Iwama, 2006). However, one of the main difficulties in understanding such key terms is the variety of ways in which culture, ethnicity, minority ethnic groups and cultural competence are defined (Dillard et al, 1992; Fitzgerald, 1997; Awaad, 2003; Purden, 2005; O'Shaughnessy & Tilki, 2006). The lack of agreement on a definitive definition contributes to confusion and creates inconsistencies, when we attempt to explore

and research cultural and ethnic concepts in relation to cultural awareness and sensitivity within professional practice. Therefore to promote
clarity within this chapter, the following definitions have been adopted.

Culture

Wells and Black (2000:279) state that 'culture refers to a set of values,
beliefs, traditions, norms, artefacts and customs that is shared by a
group or society'; whilst, Hasselkus (2002:42) defines culture as 'the
patterns of values, beliefs, symbols, perceptions and learnt behaviours
shared by members of a group and passed on from one generation to
another'. Both these definitions highlight a common set of values,
beliefs, perceptions, views and patterns of behaviour that members of
a cultural group subscribe to and uphold as important, meaningful and
of value.

What is perceived as significant is specific to that particular cultural
group and may not be shared by the majority population or the wider
society in which they live (Lim, 2001; Hunt, 2007). However, culture is
not static but is evolving and dynamic, so assumptions made about any
cultural group, and their responses and reactions to any given situation
or set of circumstances, may change and alter with time (Awaad, 2003;
Chaing & Carlson, 2003).

Understanding the term 'culture' in its widest context, is the beginning of appreciating its significance and importance. Indeed culture
can mean many things to different people and can include not only
difference in race and ethnicity, but also music, literature, food, fash-
ion, values, lifestyles and daily practices (Iwama, 2006). Dyke (1998:68)
defines culture as 'a shared system of meanings that involves ideas, concepts and knowledge which include the beliefs, values and norms that
shape standards and rules of behaviour as people go about their everyday life'.

This latter definition prompts us to look beyond limited perspectives
and to consider the possibility that two ethnically diverse individuals
socialised within a common community or society may still adopt the
same set of values, ideals and principles, for example the importance
of freedom of speech and personal choice. Lim and Iwama (2006) warn
against the dangers of racial assumptions and stereotypes that arise as
a consequence of viewing culture within such narrow limits. They challenge us to be mindful of the socio-cultural conditioning that occurs
and the impact that communities and societies have in influencing our
attitudes, values, priorities, principles, behaviours and practices.

Ethnicity

The term ethnicity, as adopted by the Commission for Race Equality
and detailed within the Office for National Statistics Census categories

(ONS, 2001), is a cultural concept that is shared by a group which has a common religious belief, genealogy, language, culture or shared traditions. This term is used to refer to a group of individuals who have shared racial origins, cultural norms and language that are ethnically rooted but not governed by nationality.

The term minority ethnic group is defined by Wells and Black (2000:282) as 'a group of persons who, because of their physical or cultural characteristics, are singled out from others in the society in which they live, for differential and unequal treatment and who regard themselves as objects of collective discrimination'. These specific individuals are distinct from the majority population due to their racial origin, cultural background and shared beliefs and, as such, are treated differently and with less regard. The consciousness of being an ethnic minority or being 'different' is reinforced as they experience incidents of overt and covert discrimination and prejudice (Lim, 2001).

In a study of undergraduate occupational therapy students at Brunel University conducted by the author, first year occupational therapy students were encouraged to explore issues of ethnicity, race, culture, health and well-being (Lim, 2004). Within the study, the majority of white English students mentioned that they felt uncomfortable with the concepts and struggled to identify their own ethnicity. In contrast, students belonging to minority ethnic groups (Asian, Black Caribbean and African) did not express the same difficulties. They mentioned that issues relating to their ethnicity, race and difference were frequently reinforced within their daily lives, through experiences of discrimination and prejudice.

The white English students within the study specifically mentioned that they had never thought about themselves in terms of their ethnicity and roots, and therefore found the task of identifying their ethnicity 'difficult' (Lim, 2004). In fact, one of the key questions arising from the study is whether being a member of a minority ethnic group, and having experienced racial discrimination, both reinforces and raises your consciousness of who you are, where you have come from and where and if you belong.

Cultural competence

Cultural competence which is identified as a goal of achieving culturally sensitive and appropriate practice, is defined as 'an awareness of, sensitivity to, and knowledge of the meaning of culture, including a willingness to learn about cultural issues, including one's own bias' (Dillard et al, 1992:722). This highlights the need for a willingness to undertake personal reflection of our own attitudes, biases and presumptions, as well as a desire to acquire knowledge and skills, if we are to be more culturally aware and sensitive. Cultural competence cannot be achieved by undertaking a course of study or an examination and then ticking a box that says we are now culturally competent. It requires a continuous and ongoing process that includes (Wells & Black, 2000; Lim, 2001):

- developing self-awareness;
- amassing a cultural knowledge base;
- knowing how to access relevant information;
- learning the skills to interact with others with sensitivity and respect;
- actively developing appropriate practice;
- incorporating sensitive strategies and negotiation skills to accommodate the needs of the individual;
- evaluating performance and outcomes appropriately.

Context

The UK is becoming increasingly multicultural and diverse. The Office for National Statistics census (ONS, 2001) indicated a total of 58.7 million people in the UK and of these 8%, or 4.7 million, are from minority ethnic groups; and this figure is predicted to continue to grow over the next decade. These statistics might not initially appear significant, however within London, 29% or over one in four of the population, are from minority ethnic groups. In some boroughs, such as Brent, Newham and Tower Hamlets, minority ethnic groups actually make up more than 50% of the population (Kings Fund, 2003). The trend towards increased diversity is not limited to London but is reflected in other regions and cities around the country, such as Glasgow, Leicester, Manchester and Bradford, where minority ethnic groups make up a significant proportion of the local population (ONS, 2001).

An examination of the current European context also raises several important issues. The growth of the European Union with a total now of 23 European member states, has resulted in a much larger common market. This has enhanced the freedom and opportunity to travel, live and work right across Europe and consequently many European countries have noted a more diverse social, cultural and ethnic population mix. Such population changes and greater diversity reinforce the need for health and social care professionals to be more aware, sensitive and competent in practising in culturally safe ways, as reflected in the current national policies and legislation.

National concerns and policies

There is a distinct need to respond to a changing and a diverse population. Public and private organisations and services are required to abide by existing national policies, guidelines and legislations that support the need to embrace diversity, tackle discrimination and promote inclusion and cultural sensitivity (CRE, 2002; Race Relation Amendment Act, 2002). High-profile cases, like the Stephen Lawrence (Lord MacPherson, 1999) and David Bennett (Blofeld, 2003) inquiries highlight the impact of institutional racism, poor levels of care, discriminatory treatments and the worrying state of public services in responding to racial discrimination, reflecting a national and societal attitude of indifference towards issues of racism and prejudice. The Macpherson Report (1999:4262-i) defined institutional racism as:

> A collective failure of an organisation to provide an appropriate and professional service to people because of their colour, culture or ethnic origins. It can be seen or detected in processes, attitudes and behaviours which amount to discrimination through the unwitting prejudice, thoughtlessness and racist stereotyping which disadvantages minority ethnic people.

Institutional racism may be both overt and covert, and public services and organisations like the police, health services, social care and education may be guilty of not addressing incidence of discrimination and racism.

Within health and social care the need to ensure culturally sensitive and safe practice is further reinforced by some worrying current statistics. The recent Healthcare Commission Census (DOH, 2005) report into mental health services indicated that black and minority ethnic (BME) service users/clients encountered:

- greater involvement of the police in their referrals;
- higher rates of physical restraint and control;
- greater likelihood of detention under the Mental Health Act (1983);
- less access to talking and psychological therapies.

National consciousness and recognition of the scale of the problem have led to governmental commitment to take action and address issues of race equality, discrimination and cultural competence within health and social care. Specific targets and provisions have been outlined within such policy documents as the National Service Frameworks (DOH, 1999), National Health Service Plan (DOH, 2000), Race and Equality in Mental Health Consultation (DOH, 2003) and the Social Exclusion Unit Report (Office of the Deputy Prime Minister, 2004). These various government policies have focused on such professional practice issues as client-centred practice, involving service users and their carers in intervention planning and providing culturally sensitive care, thereby ensuring that minority ethnic groups have the opportunities to access services they need and when they need them.

Professional culture

Within the wider context, culture can also represent organisation or profession values and structures (Carroll & Quijada, 2004). Each profession, physiotherapy and occupational therapy, can be said to possess its own cultural identity, consisting of shared values, beliefs, codes of practice and socialised behaviours. Members within these professions have been professionally trained and conditioned acquiring the cultural language, core values, priorities and habits of their particular profession (Iwama, 2004; Lim, 2005). These professional perspectives and attitudes have a significant impact on how these managers and clinicians interact, relate, behave and provide treatment.

However, before examining the potential impact that professional culture may have on practice, we need to unravel the cultural roots of each profession. An examination of the origins of both occupational therapy and physiotherapy indicates that they have evolved from a western socio-cultural context and have naturally adopted philosophies, values and principles that characterised these contextual influences. The professional values and principles of personal autonomy, function, independence, doing and active engagement, which are symbolic of western socio-culture context, have been reflected within the core values and concepts of both professional groups (Noronen & Wikstrom-Grotell, 1999; Lim & Iwama, 2006), with the presumption that these core values are representative of the priorities and interest of the clients receiving care and treatment. However we need to question if these core values and principles actually resonate with the diverse priorities and needs of the individuals we meet within our practice.

The assumption that professional core values rooted within the western socio-cultural origins of both physiotherapy and occupational therapy are universally shared and equally esteemed by our clients in practice, irrespective of their socio-cultural conditioning and contextual difference is short-sighted (Lim, 2005). Indeed as both occupational therapy and physiotherapy increase in popularity globally and more individuals have the opportunity to train and receive these modes of treatment, the need to examine the clinical utility and cultural appropriateness of existing professional values and approaches in health provision becomes even more critical (Iwama, 2004). How we respond and address individual and contextual differences in striving for culturally safe and appropriate assessments and treatment becomes an even greater priority (Gray & McPherson, 2005).

An essential step in addressing cultural safety is to recognise the impact that professional values, principles and cultures have in dictating how we communicate, assess, treat and provide services that are culturally sensitive and inclusive (Lim & Iwama, 2006). Each profession has its own cultural framework and philosophical and practice emphasis, reflected within its existing professional standards (Watson, 2006). These standards influence how the therapist views and perceives the specific needs and requirements of their individual client (Purden, 2005; Hunt, 2007).

The examination of the existing practice standards and literature within occupational therapy has indicated a notable shift in focus over the last decade, away from viewing the individual as a 'patient' to regarding them as valued clients and consumers of services (COT, 2005). Increasingly clients, carers and service user groups are consulted on several aspects of occupational therapy professional strategy, policy and treatment delivery (COT, 2006). This move away from a paternalistic view of the client as a passive recipient of care to one who is interested in being consulted and wants to be engaged as an equal partner is a significant change and challenge (Sumsion, 2004). Central to this new perspective is recognition that the client possesses the expert knowledge, power and resource to influence and determine positive changes within their own health and life experiences. The client is regarded rightly as an equal partner within his own treatment process, possessing valuable personal knowledge and unique lived experiences (Lim, 2005; COT, 2006). The shift in priority and perspective in viewing the individual client and their family and carers as central figures in all aspects of their treatment process has led to a more inclusive, empowering treatment experience for the individual concerned. This is, however, only a start and the profession needs to continually do more.

An examination of the Chartered Society of Physiotherapists (2005) Core Standards of Physiotherapy Practice highlights that the term 'patient' as opposed to 'client' is preferred and adopted as representing the treatment recipient. This choice of term, symbolic of the core values of the physiotherapy profession and its predominant biomedical influences and approaches, underpins its practice and service delivery (Hunt, 2007). Coward and Ratanakul (1999) describe how biomedicine has its own cultural values, principles and systems that both restrict and dictate the practice and priorities of the physiotherapy profession. Does this preference in viewing the individual as a 'patient' represent how the individual is regarded by the profession and clinical practitioners alike and how consultations and treatment will be organised, prioritised and decided upon?

Despite its professional standards of encouraging partnership (CSP Standards, 2005), does the physiotherapy profession still regard the individual as a passive recipient of treatment to be worked upon and intervened with? Indeed viewing the individual as 'patient' may limit the extent to which physiotherapists may feel the need to consult and address the diverse needs of their patients, if they believe that they are providing and delivering what they perceive as the 'best' and most clinically effective treatments (Lee et al, 2006; Hunt, 2007).

Professional practice, however, cannot be delivered in isolation and we need to be mindful of the wider context of political agendas, national policies, organisational priorities and cultural and professional standards that influence our treatment focus and service delivery (Davies & Nutley, 2000). Effective and quality professional practice requires an awareness of the diverse political, economic, social, national, organisational and professional agendas (Kronenberg et al, 2004) and, further, a response to the individual cultural traits and priorities of clients we encounter within our practice (Mandy et al, 2004). Indeed the impact of professional culture on clinical practice may be experienced at two levels: firstly the impact professional culture has on the quality and appropriateness of clinical treatment and care services experienced by the individual client and their family; secondly the delivery of a seamless and integrated professional service (Lim, 2005).

To ensure the client receives the most effective and culturally appropriate treatment, partnerships and negotiations need to occur between the practitioner, the client and may also include their carers (Sumsion, 2004; Purden, 2005). However genuine partnership cannot occur unless the goals of assessments and treatment are clear and transparent to the client and their carers. Practitioners immersed within their own professional culture, values, language, procedures and techniques must work at explaining and clarifying their treatment goals and processes in order for the totally unprofessionalised client to be fully included and involved in influencing the care they receive (Ells & Caniano, 2002; Lim, 2005). Failure to do so will consign the individual to be a passive recipient of care, to be treated, told what to do and remain as a lesser partner within the professional–patient relationship.

Practitioners need to strive for inclusive practice processes where goals, reasons for action, treatment options and potential consequence are openly explored and discussed to elicit the best and most appropriate intervention. The valued individual must be treated as a client entitled to information, choice and empowered to influence their own care and not merely invited to be involved in the treatment process when decisions have already been made and plans conceived (Lim, 2005; Purden, 2005). Without this transparency, open dialogue and sharing of power, how can the client and their carers be fully included in discussing, negotiating and stating their preference and influencing their treatment needs? This commitment will take more time and energy, but is critically important in ensuring meaningful, culturally safe and effective treatments (Hunt, 2007).

Within the area of inter-professional working, issues of professional ideology and priorities can be a potential stumbling block in terms of multidisciplinary working and effective clinical practice. Professional cultures and values may create tensions between the respective professions and we may be guilty of stereotyping and discriminating against another professional group to the detriment of effective multidisciplinary team working (Carroll & Quijada, 2004; Mandy et al, 2004). An illustration of this was experienced in the integration of health and social services in a community mental health team in which the author had previously been a member. Although integration on the surface seemed a good and straightforward idea in terms of ensuring a much more effective, seamless and efficient service for clients, the reality was quite different.

Despite policy initiatives and incentives to integrate teams and services, the philosophical and professional differences between health and social services, with their own distinct cultural values and structures, created major difficulties (DOH, 1999, 2001). Both sides within the new integrated team were initially pulled further apart due to professional anxiety and an unwillingness to accept the other's views, perspectives and ways of working. Multidisciplinary working in this instance was severely affected and it was only through an extended process of examining differing professional values, culture, team building and a resultant cultural shift, that the team was eventually able to function effectively as an integrated service. Purden (2005) highlights that successful partnerships within teams involve members understanding both their own role, that of others within the wider team, the common ground that exists and the boundaries that need to be respected. Indeed, without recognising, respecting and addressing the fundamental issues of professional values and cultural differences within teams, the delivery of effective, quality and culturally appropriate services would remain a distant goal.

Cultural issues and professional practice

The rich diversity and vibrancy of a multicultural UK increases the likelihood that as health and social care professionals we will meet individuals from cultures and ethnic groups that are different from our own. How we prepare, interact and respond to each individual becomes even more essential, as we strive to be more culturally aware and sensitive to the needs of those we see within our own practice (O'Shaughnessy & Tilki, 2006).

The fluid and evolving nature of culture may, however, reduce the accuracy of information we gather in preparation for meeting the client we are about to interview or assess. The initial gathering of information, although valuable, must be verified and supplemented by information gained from the client, as she will provide the best reference point in terms of her cultural and ethnic beliefs, needs and preferences. The process of culturally sensitive care is dependent upon an appreciation of the richness that defines each culture and contributes to each individual's identity, therefore, the ability to acknowledge and affirm the values and experiences of our clients is crucially important (Lim, 2001; Purden, 2005).

Recognition of the need to be culturally sensitive and competent is reflected within the respective practice standards outlined by both the College of Occupational Therapists (COT) and the Chartered Society of Physiotherapists (CPS). The COT Code of Ethics and Professional Conduct (Standard 3.2.1, 2005:9) states that:

> Occupational therapy personnel shall be aware of and sensitive to cultural and lifestyle diversity. They shall provide services that reflect and value these societal characteristics. Occupational therapy personnel shall not discriminate unlawfully and unjustifiably against clients or colleagues.

This standard clearly indicates the duty required of occupational therapists to take into account the diversity of needs and perspectives of their clients/patients in all aspects of health provision.

Similarly the Chartered Society of Physiotherapy (Standard 1.1, 2005:3) within Core Standards of Physiotherapy Practice, states that:

> Physiotherapists need to respect and respond actively to every patient as an individual. The physiotherapists should consider the patient's social, occupational, recreational, economic commitments, culture, race, gender, sexual orientation, religion, disability, age, beliefs, values, abilities and mental well being.

This standard clearly indicates recognition of the importance and value ascribed by the professional physiotherapy society in support of individualised and patient-focused treatments.

Although both statements highlight the importance and commitment placed by both professional bodies in support of cultural awareness, sensitivity and competence in practice, it must not be presumed that all managers, practitioners or students are aware of these standards or are implementing such standards within their daily practice. Indeed the process of translating standards and guidelines into everyday practice and ensuring that clinicians and students have the required awareness, knowledge and skills and commitment to implement them is far from straightforward (Dogra, 2004; Mandy, 2004).

A preliminary enquiry conducted recently by the author with a selection of nurses, social workers, physiotherapists and occupational therapists both within academia and clinical practice indicated some interesting findings and some clear disparities between the respective groups. When questioned if they felt it was important to be culturally aware and sensitive to the diverse needs of patients/clients, the response from all the individuals was affirmative. Participants also mentioned that they were aware that cultural sensitivity and competent practice were highlighted within their respective Codes of Professional Practice and Standards. However some professional groups struggled to identify and detail what the standards and guidelines actually required of them in practical terms and therefore were not able to make clear links between the standards identified and the actual educational or practice processes of implementing these standards effectively.

Education and curriculum

The majority of educators within the same enquiry mentioned that the issues of cultural awareness and sensitivity were highlighted within their curricula standards and course requirements, in responses to the requirement laid out within the respective professional core standards. However, they were less able to physically identify detailed aspects within which these issues were being addressed with the respective modules and actual teaching sessions. Distinct differences were noted between the various academic courses with some professional programmes addressing the area of cultural awareness, diversity, sensitivity and competence much more comprehensively than others.

The more effective courses required students and educators themselves to examine their own personal values and beliefs, explore diverse socio-cultural perspectives of health, well-being and illness, confront issues of racism, discrimination and prejudice and examine alternative healthcare approaches, utilising culturally sensitive procedures, complex and diverse case examples and culturally safe practice. Other courses appeared to adopt a more tokenistic view, looking merely at equal opportunities and tackling cultural issues if they arose in conversations with the students. This disparate approach is unsatisfactory and a more consistent and wholehearted approach is necessary if we are to positively address issues of cultural sensitivity and competence within current health and social care training courses (Dogra, 2004).

The variations in quality and depth in confronting issues of cultural awareness, sensitivity, discrimination etc. across the respective professional courses is of a great concern when one considers that these students would eventually be working interprofessionally and as professional practitioners. Purden (2005) supports the need for greater interprofessional training, highlighting the benefits of students being exposed to the diverse cultures, values and ideologies of other professional groups. They would also benefit from the opportunity to examine a more comprehensive spectrum of cultural perspectives and experiences.

Lee et al (2006) suggest that practitioners need to acquire culturally sensitive interview skills, culturally specific assessments and examine their existing treatment strategies in working with multicultural client groups; indeed the best environmens for students to both understand the complexity of cultures that exist within teams and the impact that cultural diversity has on practice is the clinical setting. Students who may question the relevance and need to be culturally aware and competent are left with little doubt about its importance once they have experienced the clinical realities of working with an extremely diverse population. Indeed educators, students and practitioners alike must be convinced of the importance of culturally sensitive and competent practice and its impact on effective and quality daily practice (Bennett et al, 2007).

Promoting cultural awareness and competency

The ability to be culturally aware and sensitive to the needs of those we serve is central to providing client-centred practice and promoting partnership between the patient and the professional. However the process of becoming aware of the needs of others begins with a process of self-reflection; examining our own cultural and ethnic influences, which impact upon our values, beliefs and perceptions of self and others. Only through personal examination of our own attitudes, values, assumptions and beliefs may we be able to identify our prejudices towards those we encounter in our practice and how to positively overcome these issues (McGruder, 2003; Reynolds & Lim, 2005).

Our personal values and social norms directly impact upon how we relate and respond to others; Gross (2001:351) defined value as 'a sense of what is desirable, good and worthwhile'. That is, what we consider important influences, what we place value in and how we may prioritise any given situation or set of circumstances. What is important to a professionally socialised and conditioned practitioner will not necessarily be of any importance to the next person. In fact we may inadvertently impose our own values, beliefs and prejudices on our clients and their carers (Hunt, 2007), dictating what is important, a priority or beneficial. The danger of presuming that we know what is most beneficial for our clients becomes all too apparent when they become noncompliant, de-motivated, disgruntled or simply absent from treatment (Lim, 2001).

Assumptions made without verification can also result in misinterpretation and misunderstanding. Gross (2001) identifies assumptions as acts or instances of accepting without proof things that are inherent in the attitudes that we hold towards others. Although making assumptions is unhelpful, doing so may assist us in coping and making sense of the huge volume of social information we encounter (Wetherell, 1996; Lee et al, 2006). Instead of processing information relating to each individual, we categorise them as members of homogeneous social groups (e.g. female, black, lawyers) so that our thinking and recall is simplified and manageable. The drawback is that our assumptions and perceptions of others may become accepted as true and reliable and such misrepresentations can be further reinforced by the mass media, which portrays members of certain groups in highly stereotypical ways (Reynolds & Lim, 2005).

The stereotypes we hold can also become self-fulfilling prophecies; for example, if we perceive all older people as passive, inactive and needing help, we may inadvertently encourage the very behaviour that we have anticipated (Reynolds & Lim, 2005). A key characteristic of stereotyping is that a single piece of information about an individual (such as age, gender or race) generates inferences about all other aspects of that person, including their personality, interests, aspirations and so on (Levy et al, 1998). Unexamined assumptions about members of other groups may ultimately contribute to discriminatory practices, as well as perpetuating myths and simplified perceptions.

Further, the perspectives, stereotypes and attitudes that we hold may be grounded in unexamined assumptions that members of a certain group are lazy, secretive or violent. Henley and Schott (1999:51) define attitude as 'a settled opinion or way of thinking, which is reflected in presenting behaviour'. These attitudes may be influenced by accepted norms within society that determine what attitudes and behaviours are considered to be acceptable, legitimate and what may be deemed to be deviant. Henley and Schott (1999) propose that the way we think of or perceive others, has a direct impact upon our actions, responses and behaviours towards them. How we communicate, show regard, afford time and respect the opinions of others is influenced by our attitude.

The time invested in understanding how others view, understand and interpret their own experiences can enhance cultural awareness and sensitivity. Lim and Iwama (2006) support the need for health professionals to acknowledge that different ethnic or cultural groups may have different ideas and interpretations of what influences health and well-being, alternative treatment options and the validity of diverse solutions in restoring one's health and well-being. Insight gained from these differing perspectives would enhance the quality of the professional–client relationship and also reduce potential areas of misunderstanding and misinterpretation. Helman (2007) also challenges us to be mindful of the broad cultural differences in viewing the importance of the individual self, the role of the family and the wider community. This supports the view held by Iwama (2003) that a failure to regard or respect such differences may lead to inappropriate and unsatisfactory treatment that may have little impact or therapeutic value.

Structured opportunities must be organised for students and practitioners to explore local community resources, ethnic and cultural facilities, through active community liaison, partnerships, exploratory research and spending time working with non-statutory services that are closely linked with supporting diverse communities and ethnic groups (Lim, 2005; Purden, 2005). There should be further opportunities for students and practitioners to examine and discuss their personal values, beliefs, bias and perspectives with the aim of enhancing personal awareness, insight and broadening cultural knowledge.

Exercise to promote personal awareness

A process of personal reflection and understanding of our own values, perspectives and prejudices is an essential starting point. The following exercise (Box 6.1), is designed to promote self-awareness in students and practitioners alike. It can be undertaken individually, in pairs or within a larger group.

Box 6.1 Personal and cultural awareness

This exercise provides an opportunity to explore issues relating to your own ethnicity, culture, beliefs and perceptions. Begin this exercise on your own and then, if possible, discuss your answers with a partner or within a small group.

1. How would you describe yourself in terms of your ethnicity and culture?
2. Does this view or perception of yourself influence your sense of identity? If so, how?
3. What are the common views and perceptions within your own culture around the value and importance of independence, personal autonomy, doing and choice?
4. What are the common views within your own culture around what factors contribute to an individual's health and well-being?
5. What habits, behaviours or rituals do you adopt when you are not feeling well and trying to get better? Why have you adopted them?
6. How important are beliefs, customs, spirituality or religion to you when you are unwell or in need of help?
7. Do you recall any clinical situations when you felt that the client's beliefs, identity, culture or ethnicity impacted upon his presentation, health and well-being, behaviour and recovery?
8. Identify one belief, ethnic group, culture or custom that you are unfamiliar with. Research this in relation to the areas of health, illness and well-being. Examine the possible implications of your findings to clinical practice. Examples could include: Rastafarians, Acupuncture, Christian healing, cultural attitudes and perspectives on physical touch, Indian perspectives on mental health, Seven Day Adventist dietary patterns, five pillars of Islam, cultural expressions of pain, etc.

How did you find the exercise above?
Did you experience any difficulty in identifying your own ethnic and cultural identity; if so why do you think this was the case?
What cultural insights or variations have you derived from your examination and discussion?
Did any of your answers to the above questions surprise you?

Cultural competence within the treatment process

The treatment process is perceived to begin with the first contact we have with the client, and continues through the stages of interview, assessment, intervention, evaluation and, if appropriate, discharge. However in reality the process begins well before the first face-to-face contact with the client. On receiving a referral, the therapist begins to gather relevant information about the individual, which will allow her to appreciate the situation and circumstances that the client is experiencing. In terms of a diverse client, this process should include awareness of the ethnic background, language spoken by the client and whether translation services are required.

Greetings and introductions

Preparation for meeting the client requires that we consider how we should address the client appropriately. This first contact provides a clear indication of how much we value the client, through the time and effort made to acknowledge and pronounce his/her name correctly and appropriately. It is important to take notice that there are different naming systems in the world, and that we may unintentionally offend our client if we do not adopt the appropriate mode of address (Henley & Schott, 1999). Checking the forename and surname and ensuring that our pronunciation is correct, is a small but significant gesture of respect. Our names reinforce our sense of self and identity, and are crucial to the development of our self-image, self-esteem and sense of belonging. We must not assume that the individual we meet would like to be addressed by his first name or that we are being too formal by not doing so. The most simple and effective way to ensure accuracy is to ask the client how he would like to be acknowledged (Reynolds & Lim, 2005).

Assessment

When working with culturally diverse clients, it is critical to ensure that the assessments and interventions proposed are both clinically effective and culturally appropriate. The limitations of utilising standardised assessments and outcome measures that are constructed within a totally different socio-cultural context, become apparent when the terms or language use within the assessment create greater confusion (Lim & Iwama, 2006). An example of this is reflected with a standardised assessment used within a mother and baby unit, which requires patients to indicate the last time they felt 'blue'. This term, although understood by individuals educated with a British or American context, results in difficulties in comprehension for an individual client within a different context (Reynolds & Lim, 2005). Steps must be taken to ensure that all questions are phrased appropriately, in order to elicit an accurate response from the client. The majority of assessment tools used by both physiotherapists and occupational therapists have been created and developed in the west and were often designed in conjunction with western models of practice (Iwama, 2003). Their effectiveness when used with a culturally and ethnically different client group may therefore be far more limited or valid.

Communication

Communication is essential to the treatment process and ensuring that interactions are clear and accurate is critical. Communicating with the client becomes more difficult if we are unable to speak the same language (Purden, 2005). When attempting to engage the services of interpreters we must ensure that we enlist the help of interpreters who speak the correct language or dialect. It would be naïve to assume that all individuals from a particular ethnic background, cultural group or country speak the same language. It would, for example, be presumptuous to assume that all people of Chinese origin speak Cantonese or that all individuals from Nigeria speak Yoruba.

Most health and social service departments have access to a professional interpreting and translating service and, where possible, trained professional interpreters who are familiar with medical terminology should be used. It is crucial that the client's responses are translated accurately, rather than interpreted according to what the interpreter perceives the client is trying to say, or what the interviewer may want to hear. It can be problematic, where an interpreter cannot be found and a family member is required as a last resort to undertake the translation. What the client is saying in response to a question must be translated accurately and without any form of editing that may derive a desired outcome for the relative as opposed to the actual client (Lim, 2001).

Some health terms may not exist or cannot be translated directly into the client's own language, and therefore the process of communicating becomes more difficult. The word 'stress' for example does not have a direct translation in the Chinese language; therefore it would be difficult try to gather from a Chinese speaker if he is feeling stress. It may be easier to ask about the symptoms of stress, such as poor sleep, loss of appetite, lack of energy, headaches or back pains. Indeed within some cultures, the description of somatic symptoms may be a more culturally acceptable way of presenting and communicating psychological distress and ill health (Helman, 2007).

Treatment

Consideration must be given to cultural and ethnic factors when planning interventions, by examining specific areas of practice and considering if they can be altered in order to accommodate the individual values and needs of the client. Efforts must be made to ensure that cultural sensitivity is promoted in all aspects of the intervention process (Lim, 2001). For example, when faced with clients who are Muslims or Orthodox Jews within a cookery group, a first step is to ensure that the food is halal or kosher. Care must also be taken to ensure that the equipment and utensils to be used have not been previously contaminated by having been used to prepare non-halal or kosher food. It is not sufficient in this instance to assume that because the equipment or utensils have been cleaned and washed that they are suitable for use. Individuals from these religious groups will not be able to engage and participate in cookery sessions if this is overlooked.

When treatment involves physical contact or manipulation of the individual patient, it may be assumed that as the patient is willingly attending treatment, they are therefore comfortable or consenting to be touched or handled without reservations. Gender and cultural norms around physical contact and appropriate touch must be clarified and not assumed. Regard for the person's privacy and preference, and having a therapist of the same gender to provide the therapy must be considered (Lee et al, 2006) in respect of the client's wishes.

When undertaking activities of personal care, it is important to note, for example, that African, African Caribbean and Asian individuals have different hairs and skin types, which require specialised care products. These may include coconut oil for hair grooming or specific formulated skin moisturisers. Provision must be made for catering for these needs. It may also be appropriate for the occupational therapists to master the art of putting on a 'sari', 'shalwar kameez' or 'hijab' so that dressing practice for an Asian client is adapted to accommodate appropriate clothing (Lim, 2001). Indeed, client-centred practice, a virtue of both physiotherapy and occupational therapy, is only achievable through respectful partnerships and the full appreciation and understanding of each individual's need, experiences, circumstances and wider socio-cultural context. Genuine commitment to client-centred care must be fostered by a continuous process of engaging with the clients, understanding their values and responding to their needs (Hunt, 2007).

Evaluation and outcome measurement

Outcome measurement has gained immense importance in light of the Department of Health's (UK) pursuit of clinical governance and evidence-based practice (DOH, 2001). Much attention has been focused on evidencing practice in fulfilling the government's targets highlighted within the National Health Service Plans and National Service Frameworks (Cusack & Sealey-Lapes, 2000; DOH, 2001). In the relentless pursuit of evidence-based practice, however, practitioners should not lose sight of whose outcomes they are actually measuring and whose health they are trying to promote. The danger is that it may be assumed that the client's and professional's interest and needs are the same. The client's needs may be left unmet, while practitioners attempt to meet the competing demands to evaluate and evidence their interventions and approaches.

The current emphasis and pressure to evidence practice and the use of standardised assessments to evaluate interventions raises several questions for those providing culturally sensitive care. These include what measures are being used to ascertain outcomes and results? Have they been designed for a culturally different client group? Are these assessments and measures therefore culturally appropriate when applied to different groups of individuals? Indeed the extensive promotion of standardised assessments to achieve clinical effectiveness may be flawed if the measures are selected without due care.

As previously highlighted, the majority of standardised assessments have been developed in conjunction with existing models of practice and largely constructed along western socio-cultural norms and may be limited in their appropriateness in use with a client from a different socio-cultural context (Iwama, 2003). Such measures must be adapted appropriately when used with diverse clients and supplemented with additional qualitative reporting and narratives from the client. We need to adopt an attitude of interest, active listening, exploring, explaining and clarifying, and eventual negotiation and agreement with the client (Lim & Iwama, 2006).

The use of exploratory models and a commitment to listen to the individual's narrative, acknowledge his experience and understand his concerns, is essential to this process (Mattingly & Garro, 2000). We must refrain from fitting the client into what we have already constructed, but must be truly client focused in looking at their goals and tailoring our evaluations to arrive at valid measures of the client's performance and function.

Examining clinical practice

Box 6.2 contains a list of questions that will guide you in examining and reflecting upon your own practice or clinical placement setting (see Chapter 3). Your answers to these questions may provide you with an answer to how equipped you may be in responding and in delivering culturally sensitive and competent practice.

Knowledge of our locality of practice is essential in responding to the potential needs and requirements of those we may encounter within our practice. We need to be mindful of the diversity of our local population and consider the impact that our staff mix may have upon the people who access our services. The lack of minority ethnic groups accessing our services could be a reflection of the lack of diversity within the staff group and therefore limited positive role-modelling

---

Box 6.2 Clinical reflections on practice

How aware are you of the diversity within your local clinical catchment area?
How well does your staff group/team reflect the diversity within your local catchment area?
How aware are you of the local minority ethnic community services or groups?
Do you have a resources file of the local minority ethnic and translations services?
What opportunities are available to clients/service users to access alternative treatments?
Name two initiatives that you can incorporate to improve your own practice.

(Purden, 2005). The failure to liaise with community organisations and specific minority ethnic groups may similarly limit the appeal of our services and also deny us the opportunity to be involved in valuable developmental work and partnership schemes to enhance the experiences of the client.

Cultural sensitivity and competence within clinical teams and departments can also be enhanced by the creation of a cultural resource file. This file may contain relevant information about local and community services, contact details of local translation services, immigrant services, local religious leaders and places of worship. Establishing partnerships with non-statutory and community services is also an essential step towards tackling the issue of cultural sensitivity, respecting diversity and appropriate clinical care.

Similarly, the availability of information on alternative or complementary treatments may also be a positive step forward in supporting the diverse needs of clients. The assumption that only western or medical-based treatments are the answer to all illness and health conditions is very restrictive. Servan-Schreiber (2000) supports this view within his own research by stating the limitations of western medicine and interventions in improving the quality of life and symptoms of individuals with chronic conditions. He states that, in such circumstances, complementary therapies may be much more effective and less intrusive.

Effective, quality and appropriate professional practice can only be achieved when we are responsive to the specific needs of our clients and addressing the cultural issues relating to the client is an essential component of this process. Acceptance that the interest of the client is paramount is critical towards achieving cultural sensitivity and competence. Awareness of personal values, prejudices and bias is an essential first step in ensuring respect and regard for client values, priorities, interest and needs. The acquisition of cultural knowledge and skills through education, clinical experience and continued professional development is a necessary and important process in acquiring and maintaining cultural competence in professional practice. Commitment at a professional and individual level is also critical as we continue to be mindful of how our personal and professional cultures and influences may enhance or inhibit us in providing clinically effective and culturally appropriate treatments.

If as professionals we are to provide meaningful and relevant interventions to our clients, we need to embrace the diversity that exists within our communities and to interact and respond respectfully and sensitively to the needs of our clients in pursuit of quality and best practice.

References

Awaad, T. (2003) Culture, cultural competency and occupational therapy: a review of the literature. *British Journal of Occupational Therapy* **66**(8), 356–362.

Bennett, J., Kalathil, J., Keating, F. (2007) *Race equality training in Mental Health Services in England. Does One Size Fit All?* The Sainsbury Centre for Mental Health. UK: Nuffield Press.

Blofeld, J. (2003) *Independent inquiry into the death of David Bennett*. Norwich: Norfolk, Suffolk & Cambridgeshire Strategic Health Authority.

Burnard, P. (2005) Cultural sensitivity in community nursing. *Journal of Community Nursing* **19**(10), 4–8

Carroll, J.S., Quijada, M.A. (2004) Redirecting traditional professional values to support safety: changing organisational culture in health care. *Quality Safe Health Care* **13**, 16–21.

Chaing, M., Carlson, G. (2003) Occupational therapy in multicultural contexts: issues and strategies. *British Journal of Occupational Therapy* **66**(12), 559–566.

College of Occupational Therapists (2005) *Code of Ethics and Professional Conduct for Occupational Therapists*. London: COT.

College of Occupational Therapists (2006) *Recovering Ordinary Lives. The Strategy for Occupational Therapy in Mental Health Services 2007–2017. A Vision for the Next Ten Years*. London: COT.

College of Occupational Therapists (2007) *Recovering Ordinary Lives: The Strategy for Occupational Therapy in Mental Health Services (2007–2017)*. London: COT.

Commission for Racial Equality (2002) *Strategies for Good Practice*. London: Commission for Racial Equality.

Coward, H., Ratanakul, P. (1999) *A Cross-cultural Dialogue on Health Care Ethics*. Waterloo: Wilfrid Laurier University Press.

Cusack, L., Sealey-Lapes, C. (2000) Clinical governance and user involvement. *British Journal of Occupational Therapy* **63**(11), 539–546.

Davies, H.T.O., Nutley, S.M. (2000) Organisational culture and quality of health care. *Quality in Health Care* **9**, 111–119.

Department of Health (1999) *National Service Frameworks for Mental Health*. London: HMSO.

Department of Health (2000) *National Health Service Plan*. London: HMSO.

Department of Health (2001) *NHS Plan. A Plan for Investment, a Plan for Reform*. London: HMSO.

Department of Health (2003) *Race and Equality in Mental Health Consultation Document*. London: HMSO.

Department of Health (2005) *Healthcare Commission Census*. London: HMSO.

Dillard, P.A., Andonian, L., Flores, O., Lai, L., MacRae, A., Shakir, M. (1992) Culturally competent occupational therapy in a diversely populated mental health setting. *American Journal of Occupational Therapy* **46**(8), 721–726

Dogra, N. (2004) Cultural competence or cultural sensibility comparison of two ideal type models to teach cultural diversity to medical students. *International journal of Medicine* **5**(4), 223–231.

Dyke, I. (1998) Multicultural society. In: D. Jones, S. Blair, T. Hartery and R.K. Jones (eds) *Sociology and Occupational Therapy: An Integrated Approach*. Edinburgh: Churchill Livingstone, pp. 67–79.

Ells, C., Caniano, D.A. (2002) The impact of culture on the patient-surgeon relationship. *Journal of the American College of Surgeons* **195**(4), 520–530.

Fitzgerald, M.H., Mullavey-O'Byrne, C., Clemson, L. (1997) Cultural issues from practice. *Australian Journal of Occupational Therapy* **44**(3), 1–21.

Gagliardi, P. (1990) Cultures and management training: closed minds and change in managers belonging to organizational and occupational communities. In: B.A. Turner (ed.) *Organizational Symbolism*. Berlin: de Gruyter, pp. 159–171.

Gross, R. (2001) *Psychology: the Science of Mind and Behaviour*, 4th edn. London: Hodder & Stoughton.

Gray, M., McPherson, K. (2005) Cultural safety and professional practice in occupational therapy: a New Zealand perspective. *Australian Occupational Therapy Journal* **52**(1), 34–42.

Hasselkus, B.R. (2002) *The Meaning of Everyday Occupation*. Thorofare, NJ: Slack Inc.

Helman, C.G. (2007) *Culture, Health & Illness*, 5th edn. London: Hodder & Arnold.

Henley, A., Schott, J. (1999) *Culture, Religion and Patient Care in a Multi-ethnic Society*. London: Age Concern Books.

Home Office (2002) *Race Relation Amendment Act*. Chapter 34. London: The Stationery Office.

Hunt, M. (2007) Taking culture seriously: considerations for physiotherapists. *Physiotherapy* **93**(3), 229–232.

Iwama, M. (2003) Towards culturally relevant epistemology in occupational therapy. *American Journal of Occupational Therapy* **57**(5), 582–588.

Iwama, M. (2004) Meaning and inclusion: revisiting culture in occupational therapy. *Australian Occupational Therapy Journal* **51**(1), 1–2.

Iwama, M. (2006) *The Kawa Model: Culturally Relevant Occupational Therapy*. Edinburgh: Churchill Livingstone, Elsevier.

King's Fund (2003) *London's Mental Health*. London: King's Fund.

Kronenberg, F., Algado, S.A., Pollard, N. (2004) *Occupational Therapy Without Borders Learning from the Spirit of Survivors*. Edinburgh; Churchill Livingstone.

Lee, T.S., Sullivan, G., Lansbury, G. (2006) Physiotherapists' perception of clients from culturally diverse backgrounds. *Physiotherapy* **92**(3), 166–170.

Levy, S., Stroessner, S., Dweck, C. (1998) Stereotype formation and endorsement: the role of implicit theories. *Journal of Personality & Social Psychology* **74**(66), 1421–1436.

Lim, K.H. (2001) A guide to providing culturally sensitive and appropriate occupational therapy assessments and interventions. *Mental Health Occupational Therapy Magazine* **6**(2), 26–29.

Lim, K.H. (2004) Occupational therapy in multicultural contexts. *British Journal of Occupational Therapy* **67**(1), 49–50.

Lim, K.H. (2005) Partnership, involvement and inclusion. *Mental Health Occupational Therapy* **10**(1), 22–24.

Lim, K.H., Iwama, M. (2006) Emerging models – an Asian perspective:The Kawa River Model. In: E. Duncan (ed) *Hagedorn's Foundations for Practice in Occupational Therapy*. Edinburgh: Churchill Livingstone.

Macpherson, Lord W. (1999) *The Macpherson Report*. London: HMSO Command Paper No. 4262.

Mandy, A., Milton, C., Mandy, P. (2004) Professional stereotyping and interprofessional education. *Learning in Health and Social Care* **3**(3), 154–170.

Mattingly, C., Garro, L.C. (2000) *Narrative and the Cultural Construction of Illness and Healing*. Berkeley: University of California Press.

McGruder, J. (2003) Culture, race, ethnicity and human diversity. In: E.B. Crepeau, E.S. Cohn and B.A.B. Schell (eds) *Willard and Spackman's Occupational Therapy*, 10th edn. Baltimore: Lippincott Williams and Wilkins.

Noronen, L., Wikstrom-Grotell, C. (1999) Towards a paradigm-oriented approach in psychotherapy. *Physiotherapy Theory and Practice* **15**(3), 175–184.

Office of Deputy Prime Minister (2004) *Social Exclusion and Mental Health Report*. London: Social Exclusion Unit, HMSO.

Office of National Statistics (2001) *National Census 2001*. London: HMSO.

O'Shaughnessy, D.F., Tilki, M. (2006) Cultural competency in physiotherapy: a model for training. *Physiotherapy* **93**(1), 69–77.

Purden, M. (2005) Cultural considerations in interprofessional education and practice. *Journal of Interprofessional Care* **19**(2) 224–234.

Reynolds, F., Lim, K.H. (2005) The social context of older people. In: A. McIntyre and A. Atwal (eds) *Occupational Therapy and Older People*. Oxford: Blackwell Publishing, pp. 27–48.

Servan-Schreiber, D. (2004) *Healing Without Freud or Prozac*. London: Rodale International Ltd.

Sumsion, T. (2004) Pursuing the client's goals really paid off. *British Journal of Occupational Therapy* **67**(1), 2–9.

The Chartered Society of Physiotherapy (2005) *Core Standards of Physiotherapy Practice*. London: Chartered Society of Physiotherapy Publications.

Watson, R.M. (2006) WFOT Congress. Being before doing: the cultural identity (essence) of occupational therapy. *Australian Occupational Therapy Journal* **53**(3), 151–158.

Wells, S.A., Black, R.M. (2000) *Cultural Competency for Health Professionals*. New York: The American Occupational Therapy Association Inc.

Wetherell, M. (1996) Group conflict and the social psychology of racism. In: M. Wetherell (ed) *Identities, Groups and Social Issues*. London: Sage.

7: The ethics of healthcare and multiprofessional dilemmas

David Anderson-Ford

In keeping with the aim of the text, this chapter will provide advice and discussion focused around the ethics of healthcare and multiprofessional dilemmas. In the context of this book, the term 'professional' might usefully be considered to accord with the notion of a practitioner who is able to demonstrate a high degree of competence in relation to their sphere of healthcare delivery. It is with this in mind that the Chartered Society of Physiotherapy and the College of Occupational Therapists provide detailed codes of professional practice, the core elements of which present the current summation of deep and long-standing debate concerning the ethical and legal issues underpinning best practice (COT, 2005; CSP, 2005).

With regard to the ethical aspects of professional practice in healthcare, it is useful to revisit initial definitions and concepts of what is meant by 'ethical issues'. The terms 'ethics' and 'morality' are generally considered to bear the same meaning, and, in a healthcare context tend to be used to determine a set of values concerning how men and women (in this case health professionals) ought to lead their lives – standards of conduct whose purpose is to benefit others (Pattinson, 2006). Morality, in practice, tends to concern the process of deliberation, of debate, concerning the 'rightness' or 'wrongness' of a particular issue. Usually, in a healthcare context, this concerns a situation which presents itself as a dilemma, leading to a discourse about how the dilemma might reasonably be resolved in accordance with a common understanding (if such is possible) concerning the 'best', ethically justifiable, solution.

Over the past 25 years or so, courts in the UK have been constantly challenged in relation to requests to solve some of these dilemmas. Living as we do in a rights-based society, if rights are unclear, or indeed non-existent, as has proved to be the case with many healthcare dilemmas, then the courts have been sought to provide at least an interim solution, pending potential intervention by Parliament. There are a considerable number of examples of this, but you will be well aware of some of the headline makers: the Anthony Bland case (Airedale NHS versus Bland, 1993) literally concerned matters of life and death. See also Re C (1993), a case beginning a long debate about the meaning and definition of capacity, leading to the passing of the Mental Capacity Act 1995 (United Kingdom Parliament, 1995).

It can be argued (see Seedhouse, 1998) that there are two types of ethics in a practical context: what might be termed 'everyday ethics' and, on the other hand, 'technical ethics'. Everyday ethics is not part of the intellectual and professional debate concerning professional ethics. Quite properly, everyone has an opinion and, often, is not reluctant to voice it amongst various groups of people. These discussions/ arguments tend to be prompted by some headline-grabbing dilemma, not unknown in healthcare, where such matters frequently concern life and/or death. Obvious examples include: withdrawal of treatment, genetic engineering, abortion, euthanasia and the science of in vitro fertilisation (IVF). Whilst such opinionated debates should be applauded to discourage apathy, they, more likely than not, fail the test of evidence, i.e. where is the evidence for the assertions made and/or where is the ethically based justification?

On the other hand, technical ethics, as the philosophers will inform us, concerns the attempt to design a theory which is internally coherent and which enables a person to 'act morally' (according to the particular theory arrived at), whatever the situation in life is which confronts that person – in this case, you as a health professional (Seedhouse, 1998). You will observe that technical ethics is attempting to design *a* theory, not the theory, and this (inevitably) leads to a problem when attempting to resolve professional dilemmas. You will no doubt be aware that there are a number of different schools of ethics which, although they share a common goal, that moral philosophy is a quest to understand 'good', have very different ways of viewing the process of seeking a solution.

In relation to professional practice in healthcare, two particular schools of philosophical thought are most readily apparent and, indeed, very real on a day-to-day basis. These ethical matters are not solely confined to elegant discussions in textbooks and learned journals. They are very much 'coal face' issues. Take, for example, the ethics of resource allocation within the National Health Service. Two schools of ethics are to the fore in the current debate. The first school, emanating from the work of Jeremy Bentham and John Stewart Mill in the nineteenth century is commonly known as 'utilitarianism' or 'consequentialism', sometimes referred to as 'teleology' (Bentham, 1781; Mill, 1860). Cutting through the jargon, you are likely to recognise a number of widely propounded maxims which tend to be associated with this school. For example:

- let the ends justify the means;
- the greatest happiness for the greatest number;
- maximise benefit; minimise harm.

These fine-sounding statements, containing as they do an implication that the more happiness and benefit that can be provided, the more justifiable the activity, are not without their criticisms. The first major criticism, it might be argued, concerns the fact that, if the end, i.e. goal, can be justified as 'good', then the process, procedure and practice by which that goal is reached is not as ethically important. This criticism was made most chillingly manifest at the Nuremberg war crimes trials in 1945 (Wendling, 2001). The tribunal heard evidence that medically qualified researchers had caused the death of hundreds of thousands of concentration camp inmates in the name of science. Their argument was that if the ultimate goal, e.g. benefit to human kind as a whole, was justifiable, then the sacrifice of a number of people in order to reach such a goal is ethically sustainable.

The second problem arising from the above maxims is the term 'happiness', or indeed 'benefit'. How are these terms to be defined? The answer, quite frequently, tends to be subjective. What creates happiness in one person might not in another. It is easy to see that resource allocation determinations within the NHS are frequently made on a utilitarian basis, i.e. numbers. The greater the number of people treated, the more the good aim is satisfied. The deleterious effect of this is that the more expensive a treatment, the less likely it is that it will be administered, i.e. individual needs are compromised in the name of maximising benefit (see R v Cambridge Health Authority, 1995).

The deontologist, on the other hand, sees the world very differently. Emerging from the writings of the eighteenth century philosopher Immanuel Kant, this school of thought is based on the notion of the moral imperative (Kant, 1785), i.e. that, rather than concentrating on the ends justifying the means, individuals are an end in themselves, deserving of recognition in terms of moral rights. If an individual has rights conferred upon them, then a duty and obligation arises to recognise those rights and to allow them to be asserted. In the modern day, autonomy and duty of care are the most obvious examples. Returning to the Nuremberg trials, the reader will note that the consequentialist defence foundered, i.e. a deontological view was imposed, firmly asserting that the autonomy of the individual was absolutely central to science and that, therefore, consent, what we would now term informed consent, lay at the heart of all research endeavour. What emerged from this discourse was the Nuremberg Code 1945 which now forms the fundamental basis for ethical conduct in research, although considerable refinements have now been made to the original components by the Declaration of Helsinki 1964 (World Medical Association, 2007).

Emerging from the above, and indeed, in an endeavour to create a 'road map' to begin to define 'good' in professional practice to enable your codes of practice and standards to be drafted and to provide defensible principles upon which to base day-to-day practice, the modern-day ethics of health care, certainly within a western European context, are likely to conform to five guiding principles, propounded and refined by Beauchamp and Childress (2001) and Theroux (2003).

The value of life

The Nuremberg Code echoed the consequentialist maxim 'maximise benefit; minimise harm', but this was meant in a different context, i.e.

the greater the risk to life itself in relation to any one individual, the less likely it would be that this would be professionally defensible either in practice or in relation to research endeavour. That said, the Bland Case (Airedale NHS versus Bland, 1993) is a clear expression of the dilemmas exposed in situations where further treatment appears to be futile and where withdrawal of treatment might, in certain circumstances, be justified as ethically sustainable even where death results. The courts are of the view that what is often referred to as the 'sanctity of life' is not an absolute. For example, the Doctrine of Double Effect (McIntryre, 2006) is widely known and practised throughout healthcare in terminal cases where an individual is in considerable pain. The science of the matter tells us that the application of morphine will reduce the pain, thus improving the so-called quality of life, but, as the dosage will need to be progressively increased in order to maintain the same effect, science also tells us that this will shorten the life of the individual. Modern practice finds itself able to ethically defend this situation on the basis that, in appropriate cases, i.e. at the end of the line so far as treatment is concerned (known as futility), improving the quality of a person's life can be justified to outweigh length of life. How? Because the motive for increasing the dosage is not to kill, but to improve what life is left in the context of futility. And so it was with Anthony Bland, i.e. further treatment was considered futile and that withdrawal of treatment became ethically defensible as his death would be brought about, not by the active intervention of the health professional, but by the underlying impairment which he was suffering. Thus, the ethics of the matter can be distilled down into the issue of motive. If the motive is good, i.e. the intention is beneficent, and that active assistance is not being rendered to do harm, then the good motive outweighs the bad consequence.

The above justification is by no means universally accepted (Mason and Laurie, 2005; Pattinson, 2006) and might be referred to as an example of 'soft focus ethics', i.e. it provokes an everyday ethics, emotive response, to a huge dilemma – it feels better; we can live with it. The fact is, say the critics, sanctity of life is being compromised in an avoidable way. Although it might be disguised under the blanket of withdrawal of treatment, as opposed to actively assisting death, it is the act of human agency which causes the end result, i.e. death. Since 1993, the Bland case has been frequently revisited, but remains current law and practice and is likely to so continue for the foreseeable future.

Today, the issues raised by Bland and other such cases have moved on to parallel matters, for example euthanasia. Returning to resources and the consequentialist argument for application of resources, you are reminded of the matter of QALYS, i.e. quality adjusted life years (Sutton, 2006). If resources are limited and 'the demand exceeds the supply', then how are we to prioritise in terms of access to that supply? What criteria might ethically be defended in support of person A, rather than person B or C, qualifying for the treatment? This is a particularly acute dilemma where the treatment is life saving.

Goodness or rightness

The main driver here is the notion of 'do no harm', so this again quite often concerns motive. Interestingly, therefore, harm may well result from a good motive. A fact reflected in the law where consequences could not reasonably be foreseen. Long enshrined in medical ethics have been the notions of beneficence (endeavour to benefit), nonmalfeasance (avoid causing harm) and malfeasance. The latter concerns recklessness or intent to inflict harm on an individual, i.e. the opposite of 'good' in an ethical context, and, as we know, this extreme end of ethical conduct tends to cross over into criminal law (Pattinson, 2006).

Justice or fairness

The first problem here is to recognise the almost impossible task of attempting to define terms; that said, examples from practice might usefully provide guidance. The concept of non-discrimination is embedded within the National Health Service – the cost of the treatment is not related to the wealth of the patient, although the criteria driving a waiting list may well be controversial. In research, considerable care needs to be taken with regard to the recruitment of research participants. Inclusion/exclusion criteria require explicit drafting so as not to convey the impression of wishing to be less than fair in allowing access to a research study. There are numerous examples of this, e.g. age or language restrictions (National Patient Safety Agency, 2007).

Truth-telling

A stark example of the application of the precepts of different schools of ethical thought becomes apparent here. With patients and clients, a frequent dilemma arises in relation to how much information should be imparted to them. On the one hand, the law has reasonably modest requirements in terms of a duty to impart information, if the patient so requests it. Although the modern trend is to use the term 'informed consent' and imply that the patient or client has clearly delineated rights to information, technically speaking, the law continues to support the notion of therapeutic discretion (Montgomery, 2003); it could be argued that this is, itself, a consequentialist notion. It may be explained thus: let the end justify the means. The good is to act in the best interests of the patient or the client. Thus, in some cases, it may be that imparting key elements of information to such a person would not, on the basis of therapeutic privilege, be considered in the patient's best interests; i.e. it is thought that the result would do more harm than good, contrary to the notion of beneficence.

The deontologist, on the other hand, strictly applying the notion of the moral imperative, might adopt a totally opposite stance, i.e. there is a moral obligation, a moral imperative, to tell the truth in each and every case. In the situation where the patient or client is not asking for information, the imperative might be much less clear. Is there a duty to tell in such an apparently passive situation, bearing in mind what appears below, i.e. the issue of autonomy?

Autonomy

This is often used in alternative expressions such as 'self-determination' or 'freedom to choose' and is frequently presented as the most self-evident and fundamental ethical value (Beauchamp & Childress, 2001). It is apparent that in modern day professional practice, 'patient- and client-centred' is the order of the day, as is respect for the right of the individual to give, or indeed to withhold consent. That said, perhaps matters are not as self-evident as they might at first sight appear. Human rights law, based on the European Convention of Human Rights 1950, has recognised that, where the wish to autonomously exercise a right clashes with the collective rights of a community, then a dilemma arises, i.e. what is the extent to which the rights of the individual, where there is such a conflict, should be upheld. The reader will be well aware of the public interest issue arising from confidential relationships between health professionals and patients.

A further topical issue relates to the fact that autonomy inevitably forms a central theme for an ethical framework of practice, but is solely reliant on the capacity of an individual to exercise choice. It is not the quality of the decision that is relevant here (see Re MB (Caesarean Section), 1997); it is the capacity to make a decision, even if others, indeed most other people, would consider the decision 'wrong'. The matter of capacity has taxed the courts to a considerable extent over the past two decades, both in relation to adults and children (Gillick v West Norfolk and Wisbech Area Health Authority, 1986). The case of Re C (1994) at least provided care contexts: Is the patient able to comprehend and retain the information provided? Does he or she believe it? Is the individual capable of weighing the risks on the basis of which choices may be made? This test, with the omission of the belief criterion, now forms the basis of Section 3 of the Mental Capacity Act 2005, with a further over-arching consideration (Section 2) that capacity is presumed until the contrary is demonstrated.

Ethical dilemmas are most clearly to the fore in situations where the individual either patently lacks capacity or where there is doubt as to the extent of that capacity (see Re B, 2002). Quite often a tension is created between what might be termed a paternalistic approach to the best interests of the individual and the strong promotion of the notion that, wherever possible, autonomy should be respected. Clearly, there are resource implications, based upon 'maximising throughput'; the professional might feel compromised when wishing to take more time to offer explanation, but actually being unable to spare that time because of other priorities.

Equally, where autonomy is absent, how then best to proceed, ethically and legally? The well worn term in such instances is 'best' as in 'best interests' – but what interests? And what, in the particular instance, qualifies as 'best'? You will be aware that the Mental Capacity Act 2005 (United Kingdom Parliament, 2005) has attempted to provide guidance on this matter by way of a set of criteria for consideration where relevant. These criteria (set out in Section 4 of the Act) may prove useful in the solving of ethical dilemmas in a professional context, and the reader will note that the criteria are much wider than purely 'medical' interests. Autonomy is writ large here – 'past and present wishes and feelings' S.4(6)(a) … (if known) 'beliefs and values' S.4(6)(b), together with an over-arching notion stressing encouragement to participate in decision making to the fullest possible extent. In other words, there is a strong deontological core to the statutory notion of 'best interests' which could well prove useful for more general application in terms of problem solving. Both healthcare law and ethics are littered with soundbites – phrases and maxims which might sound impressive at first hearing, but which, upon subsequent examination, prove extremely illusive in terms of meaning and substance. 'Welfare, 'need' and 'public interest' are all examples of the phenomenon, and each should be weighed carefully in the context of ethical practice (Pattinson, 2006).

Ethics in research

Another ethical dimension relating to professional practice concerns the duty placed upon the health professional to keep up to date with the latest general trends within their particular sphere of practice (CSP, 2005; COT, 2005). In order to advance this endeavour, occupational therapists and physiotherapists are frequently involving themselves in conducting or participating in research projects.

There are at least two ethics dimensions to this activity, i.e. the formulation of a research ethics proposal and also carrying out the research in an ethical manner. Both activities are subject to a certain amount of control, particularly within the sphere of the National Health Service and, increasingly, within local authorities (National Patient Safety Agency, 2007). Applications to conduct research within the National Health Service require that a National Research Ethics Services (NRES) electronic form be completed. Although the form has attracted criticism, most particularly in relation to its length (Pugsley & Dornan, 2007), it is intended to probe the same areas of enquiry referred to above in relation to the core elements of ethics in healthcare practice. It is submitted that the correct term is not 'research ethics', but rather 'ethics in research' on the basis that there is nothing special or different about these core elements. Respect for the person, autonomy, confidentiality and the duty of care (in both an ethical and legal sense) lie at the heart of the application.

There are also other elements that bear strong similarities to practice. For example, risk assessment. Bearing in mind the deontological, rather than the consequentialist, notion of risk, i.e. the greater the risk of harm, the less professionally advised or ethical the activity would be, the notion of weighing risk against benefit is a key element in the concept of duty of care. Other similarities may be noted. For example, the concept of informed consent has both ethical and legal roots – it may be argued that the choice can only be exercised realistically if sufficient information is given to enable the patient, client, or research participant to make a measured judgement. In fact, in relation to the ethics of research, the requirements are somewhat higher in terms of information giving than would actually be required within a purely legal context, where the therapeutic notion of best interests might prevail (Montgomery, 2003). Hence, in research, there is a very heavy emphasis upon the Research Participant Information Sheet (National Patient Safety Agency, 2007) which must contain a considerable amount of detailed information, but which must also be conveyed in a manner capable of being understood by the recipient.

The health professional seeking to engage in public sector research within the National Health Service or a local authority context is advised to consult not only the web site (http://www.nres.npsa.nhs.uk/rec-community/guidance/) but also crucial texts by way of guidance, for example the Declaration of Helsinki (http://www.wma.net/e/policy/b3.htm).

Illustrative case study material

Dilemma 1

You are a therapist working in an inpatient hospital unit for teenagers. A 14-year-old patient who has been admitted with a fractured arm and mild head injury asks you to promise to keep a secret. She then discloses to you that she is physically abused at home by her mother and this was the cause of her injuries. She tells you that it is the first time that she has been hurt and that she feels confident that her mother will not do it again. She tells you not to tell anyone and reminds you that you promised not to tell.

When considering this matter, you would be well advised to ask yourself the following questions:

- What are the issues?
- What should you do?
- What would you do?
- How would you feel?

The above serves as a useful illustration of the tension between a deontological approach to professional dilemmas, as set against a consequentialist approach. Taking the notions of respect and duty of care as the principal issues, then confidentiality is to be considered of primary importance in normal circumstances – the relationship between health professional and patient/client could hardly be justified without it. Thus, a strict, absolutist approach to the dilemma forces the conclusion that the information cannot be imparted because to do so would breach trust and, indeed, lead to the breaking of a promise. That said, in appropriate 'public interest' situations (reflected in ethics and law, e.g. Article 8, European Convention on Human Rights, 1950 (Human Rights Act 1998) (United Kingdom Parliament, 1998); W. v Egdell (1989)), a consequentialist justification emerges on the 'minimise harm, maximise benefit' basis. This is reflected in the general understanding of the term 'public interest', i.e. where there is the likelihood of serious harm being caused to others, then this will outweigh personal interests and rights. There is, in fact, nothing special as far as general principles are concerned about the fact that the patient is 14 years old. This could just as easily be exemplified in the context of domestic violence by one elderly protagonist against another. That said, the law of child protection (Children Act, 1989) is automatically engaged on the basis of an historical requirement that the state owes a duty of care to vulnerable persons, most particularly children and young persons.

The risk potential in the above scenario in legal terms translates into a strict requirement to breach confidentiality in the public interest, the ethical defence, as stated above, being the consequentialist notion of collective protection.

How would you feel? Probably a mixture of emotions. On the one hand, a life may well be saved; on the other hand, trust is possibly irredeemably lost. You may wish to explore the dilemma of actions potentially causing harm in one sense, maximising benefit in another by examining such cases as the Conjoined Twins Case (2001), which returns us to the motive aspects of the argument discussed above in relation to double effect. You will recall that the Conjoined Twins Case was resolved by the Court of Appeal sanctioning the surgical separation of the twins, even though one would inevitably die. The justification was twofold – one life would be saved (if the separation had not taken place, the clinical evidence was that both twins would die) and further, the motive for separation was not to end life. That would occur because of the underlying impairment.

Dilemma 2

You have been called to see a patient on an older adult ward who has an acute chest infection and is unable to maintain his airway. He is not a candidate for resuscitation, intensive care or ventilation and is at risk of dying unless he can clear the secretions. It is felt that this is an acute exacerbation and that if he survives this episode, the prognosis is good and he should return home. In spite of trying many respiratory techniques, you are unable to help him clear his airways, and it is therefore decided to perform nasopharangeal suction on the patient. He initially agrees to this invasive and very uncomfortable procedure, but after the first attempt says he cannot go through it again and begs you to stop. You know that without this treatment, he is likely to suffer a respiratory arrest and die.

- What are the issues?
- What should you do?
- What would you do?
- How would you feel?

The ethics and the law of the matter, at least initially, run not just in parallel but in a mixed stream, i.e. the autonomy of the individual with capacity is to be respected above all else, unless rights clash between individual and collective well-being as in Dilemma 1 above. Assuming that the patient retains capacity, then the autonomy of the individual to refuse treatment must be respected, a failure to recognise the importance of the notion of respect giving rise at least to the potential for a legal action based on assault and battery. This would not prevent a duty to provide sufficient information and a duty to warn the individual of the risks and consequences of withdrawing consent. In childcare law, even where the child or young person might be considered to possess Gillick Competence (Gillick v West Norfolk and Wisbech Area Health Authority, 1986) to give consent, in the vast majority of cases where such individuals have refused consent their refusal has been over-ridden, on the basis that, whilst capacity might exist to consent, it is not necessarily present to dissent due to lack of experience in terms of understanding the consequences of refusal. This of course, will not apply here, as autonomy must be respected to its fullest extent. So to repeat, capacity must be presumed unless otherwise indicated and therefore refusal must be upheld.

How would you feel? Again, a tension is revealed. Health professionals often experience the desire to exercise duty of care to its fullest extent, to save lives, to maximise benefit. There is a tendency for the wish to extend the duty of care beyond what might be considered modern parameters. Paternalism (the therapeutic desire to determine the best interests of an individual on their behalf) has tended, in the modern era, to take a back seat in favour of the deontological focus on the rights of the individual. If there is a public safety issue, which might arise for example in mental disorder cases, when deciding whether to remove a patient from section under mental health legislation with a view to potentially allowing the patient to return to the community, the health and safety of others must be weighed against the health and safety of the individual. Interestingly, and somewhat controversially, mental health law does not focus on capacity when determining whether to compulsorily detain an individual.

Dilemma 3

As a healthcare professional, you decide to undertake a course of further study which involves actively conducting research for a higher degree dissertation. You currently engage on a daily basis with patients and clients and it occurs to you that the population sample from which participants could be drawn to take part in your proposed research offers a ready made group to approach.

▪ What are the issues?
▪ What should you do?

The core of the dilemma here is potential conflict of interest. On the one hand, you are a therapist in a professional relationship with a patient or client, wherein respect and a duty of care become synonymous and automatically apply. On the other hand, but at the same time (at least in the eyes of the patient or client) you wish to conduct research, no doubt for sound and justifiable reasons. Nonetheless, as referred to above, informed consent is vitally important, both in terms of the provision of treatment, but also when inviting participation in a research project. The question has to be asked how voluntary will consent be, if given? What will happen to me if I refuse? Will treatment be withdrawn, or even will my health professional not be nice to me any more? Thus, the potential conflict of interest will need to be resolved. Otherwise, freedom of choice may become seriously compromised – not because it was intended, but because its implication had unforeseen consequences. Two suggestions for resolution may be proffered:

▪ Must these be your patients or clients? Can another group be obtained to serve the same purpose? This option is to be preferred.
▪ If not, careful attention must be paid to the information, both written and oral, communicated to the would-be participant. Adequate time for reflection, together with a clear statement that not taking part will in no way reflect on, or prejudice treatment and/or other services to which the individual is entitled, should become an integral part of the consenting process. A way of further distancing yourself from potentially compromising consent would be to use another individual to undertake the consenting process.

Chapter summary

The basic intention of this chapter has been to provide a brief introduction, via a series of triggers and widely publicised examples, to the very real ethical dilemmas likely to confront the health professional. Frequently, particularly given rapid scientific progress, there are no 'right' answers. That said we necessarily are obligated, to ourselves and others, to justify what we do, and why we do it. It's called accountability.

References

A (Children) Conjoined Twins (2001): Surgical Separation, Re (2001) Fam 147.

Airedale NHS v Bland (1993) A.C. 789.

Beauchamp, T.L., Childress, J.F. (2001) *Principles of Biomedical Ethics*. Oxford: Oxford University Press.

Bentham, J. (1781) *An Introduction to the Principles and Morals of Legislation*. Oxford. http://phi673uw.files.wordpress.com/2007/01/bentham_mills.pdf (Accessed 11th June 2008).

British Association of Occupational Therapists (2005) *The* Code *of* Ethics *and Professional* Conduct *for Occupational Therapists*. London: College of Occupational Therapists.

Chartered Society of Physiotherapy (2005) *Rules of Professional Conduct*. London: Chartered Society of Physiotherapy.

Gillick v West Norfolk and Wisbech Area Health Authority (1986) AC 112.

Kant, I. (1785) *Fundamental Principles of the Metaphysics of Morals*. Transalated by T.K. Abbott. http://philosophy.eserver.org/kant/metaphys-of-morals.txt (Accessed 14th June 2008).

Mason, J.K., Laurie, G.T. (2005) Euthanasia. In: J. Mason and R. McCall Smith (eds) *Law & Medical Ethics*. Oxford: Oxford University Press.

McIntyre, A. (2006) *Doctrine of Double Effect, Stanford Encyclopaedia of Philosophy*. http://plato.stanford.edu/entries/double-effect/ (Accessed 20th June 2008).

Mill, J.S. (1860) *On Liberty*. Oxford: Clarendon Press.

Montgomery, J. (2003) *Health Care Law*. Oxford: Oxford University Press.

National Patient Safety Agency (2007) *National Research Ethics Service Information Sheets & Consent Forms*. http://www.nres.npsa.nhs.uk/rec-community/guidance/ (Accessed 14th June 2008).

Pattinson, S.D. (2006) *Medical Law and Ethics*. London: Sweet & Maxwell.

Pugsley, L., Dornan, T. (2007) Using a sledgehammer to crack a nut: clinical ethics review and medical education research projects. *Medical Education* **41**(8), 726–728.

R v Cambridge Health Authority, ex parte B (1995) 1FLR 1055.

Re B (2002) EWHC 429.

Re C (1984) Adult: Refusal of Medical Treatment. Re (1994) 1 WLR 290.

Re MB (Caesarean Section) (1997) 8 Med LR 217 per Bultler-Sloss LJ at 224.

Seedhouse, D. (1998) *Ethics. The Heart of Health Care*. Chichester: John Wiley & Sons.

Sutton, A. (2006) Quality *Adjusted Life Years (QUALYS)* NHS National Library for Health http://www.library.nhs.uk/HealthManagement/ViewResource.aspx?resID=123545 (Accessed 14th June 2008).

United Kingdom Parliament (1998) *Schedule 1, Human Rights Act.* http://www.opsi.gov.uk/ACTS/acts1998/ukpga_19980042_en_1 (Accessed 14th June 2008).

United Kingdom Parliament (2005) *Mental Capacity Act.* http://www.opsi.gov.uk/acts/acts2005/en/ukpgaen_20050009_en_1 (Accessed 14th June 2008).

United Kingdom Parliament (2004) *Children Act.* http://www.opsi.gov.uk/acts/acts2004/ukpga_20040031_en_1 (Accessed 14th June 2008).

Theroux, J.P. (2003) *Ethics: Theory and Practice.* London: Prentice Hall.

W v Egdell (1990) 1AllER 835.

Wendling, P. (2001) The Origins of Informed Consent. The International Scientific Communication of Medical War Crimes and the Nuremberg Code. *Bulletin of the History of Medicine* **75**(1), 37–71.

World Medical Association (Revised 2007) *Declaration of Helsinki.* World Medical Association http://www.wma.net/e/ethicsunit/policies.htm (Accessed 28th August 2008).

8: Documentation and the use of the International Classification of Functioning, Disability and Health (ICF) in interprofessional working

Anne McIntyre

This chapter will explore related issues that are relevant to interprofessional working; the keeping of documentation and the use of the World Health Organization's (WHO) International Classification of Functioning, Disability and Health (ICF) (WHO, 2001). The chapter will firstly consider recent and current issues in professional documentation that relate to patients/clients/service users. The ICF will then be considered in terms of the provision of a common taxonomy, classification and framework for documentation and interprofessional practice. In addition, the potential of the recently introduced ICF core sets to facilitate interprofessional working will be explored. The term 'service user' will be used throughout this chapter as describing those individuals who use/receive health and/or social care services.

What is documentation?

Documentation within health and social care settings encompasses all aspects of information and evidence for the provision of services to service users. These can include integrated care or therapy pathways, local or national guidance and protocols; which, although important because of their influence on practice, will not be considered here. The focus of this chapter is the record keeping of information about intervention with individual service users, commonly known as care records. Not only would care records include documentation of the therapeutic involvement and intervention with a service user but would also contain any reports that may have been written as a result of interventions such as e-mails, letters, copies of telephone conversations, audio or visual recordings, digital images, notes or supervision records generated on behalf of the service user. Care records may be unique to a profession and a service or may be shared and integrated across professions and services, congruent with interprofessional and inter-agency working.

Context of documentation

The recording of interviews and the assessment of service users, as well as subsequent interventions and reports are a crucial (and legal) aspect of professional practice, which are highly valued internationally and nationally by professional bodies and employing organisations as a core competence for practice.

As the Nursing and Midwifery Council (NMC) (2007) states, record keeping is not an optional extra. However there is evidence that record keeping can be perceived as a time-consuming, low-priority and peripheral activity in comparison to face-to-face involvement with service users (Cumming et al, 2001) and not the primary consideration of practice (Wood, 2001). In extreme cases therapists have had their fitness to practise scrutinised and their licence to practise suspended by their regulatory body; for example the Health Professions Council (HPC) in the UK, citing unsafe practice due to incompetent, inadequate or missing record keeping, as well as falsification and inability to provide clear and concise records (HPC, 2007).

Even though it is considered that the quality of the records kept mirrors the quality of the intervention given, it could be argued that good documentation does not always infer good practice. Indeed, a service user is often primarily concerned about the practitioner's therapeutic expertise rather than their clerical and administrative skills (Wood, 2001; NMC, 2007). However one needs to consider that poor documentation in care records reduces the opportunity to demonstrate good as well as bad practice (Cumming et al, 2001) and can be perceived as a poor representation of the profession as a whole (College of Occupational Therapists (COT), 2006).

The accurate keeping of care records is therefore highly valued by health and social care professions because these are often the primary means of communication between interprofessional and inter-agency team members. These records document the assessment, intervention and outcome which have taken place, as well as demonstrating that risk management and legal and policy requirements have been adequately addressed.

Good documentation is critical in the decision-making process about the appropriate management for a service user, as it evidences how the assessment, diagnosis and prognosis process has informed intervention. Care records allow for appropriate continuity of care where a service user has a progressive or chronic health condition and will be seen over a prolonged period of time or when the service user is referred from one service to another. Well documented care records allow the team to identify prior clinical reasoning and intervention and to demonstrate and articulate their own. When these records are combined they provide a sound evidence base for both clinical audit and research, as it is considered that good quality records 'underpin(s) the delivery of high quality evidence based health care' (Department of Health, 2005:5).

Documentation as part of risk management

It is widely accepted that poor documentation leads to an increased risk for service users and that documentation is an integral part of risk management for organisations (Cumming et al, 2001; COT, 2006). Lack of or poor documentary evidence can lead to inappropriate discharges, poor and inappropriate decision making for intervention and in worst cases a life-threatening outcome for the service user. Where information is omitted or inadequate there is a lack of transparency and accountability of the practitioner's involvement with a service user. However, good documentation identifies that legal and policy requirements (including user consent) have been met and thus protects the practitioner (or service) from accusation of negligence or misconduct (Cumming et al, 2001). This is especially important within client-centred practice where the service user is encouraged to have choice and control of their life and therefore potentially make higher-risk decisions. Therefore, the practitioner must be able to demonstrate through their documentation that the service user was adequately supported and informed during their decision-making process (DOH, 2007a).

In 2003, the Climbié Inquiry was carried out in the UK by Lord Laming, and has had a great impact on the keeping and monitoring of care records, especially within children's services. This inquiry identified that poor documentation and monitoring of care records by health, social care and police services was a major contributory factor to the death of Victoria Climbié, aged 8, in 2000, secondary to continuous and long-term non-accidental injury. As a result of the Laming report (HMSO, 2003) it was identified that all professionals working with children should keep complete, appropriate and up-to-date records of all communications and transactions including discussions of concerns of potential deliberate harm.

Many of the Climbié Inquiry (HMSO, 2003) recommendations have been adopted by professional bodies (Chartered Society of Physiotherapy (CSP), 2005; COT 2006; NMC, 2007) and organisations as standard for care record management for all service users. Indeed even the prompt recording of non-attendance can be crucial as this can quickly identify potentially life-threatening behaviours by service users. Where service users are at risk by the actions of others or indeed where they are a potential risk for other people because of violent behaviour, the recording of this potential high risk needs to be carried out responsibly and within local policy guidelines and legal requirements. The use of a 'common language' within and across agencies (HMSO, 2003) as well as the appropriate security of information is necessary to safeguard both service user and practitioners. Regular monitoring of care records through audit by line managers (e.g. random sampling once every 3 months) is now commonplace to ensure that any risk is minimised and the relevance and currency of any potential risk is regularly reviewed.

The impact of legislation and policy on documentation

Even though the content of the records we keep is highly important, practitioners need to be mindful of other issues with documentation that relate to service users. These concerns include access to records plus the handling, management, safekeeping and disposal of records. In the UK and other countries, statute law and government policy impact on record keeping as well as local protocols and professional guidelines. Historically, when keeping care records, duty of confidentiality and user consent have been subject to common law. Current policy in the UK for example, has been strongly influenced by two key reports: the Caldicott Report (DOH, 1997) and the Audit Commission review of Health Records Services in 1999 (see Box 8.1).

In 1995, the Audit Commission in the UK undertook a study of care records within the NHS and established that these were inadequately

---

Box 8.1 Legislation, policy and government reports impacting upon record keeping in the UK

Legislation

Human Rights Act (1998)
Data Protection Act (1998)
Access to Health Records Act (1990)
Access to Health Records (Northern Ireland) Order (1993)
Freedom of Information Act (2000)
Freedom of Information (Scotland) Act (2002)

Policy

NHS Confidentiality: Code of Practice (2003)
Records Management: NHS Code of Practice (2006)
NHS Connecting for Health: Information Governance (2007)
The Care Record Guarantee: NHS Connecting for Health (2007)

Reports

Department of Health (1997) Report on the Review of Patient-identifiable Information – Caldicott Report.
Audit Commission (1999) Setting the Records Straight: A review of progress in Health Records Services.

stored, difficult to retrieve when required for service user consultation, with poor organisation of content. All of these could compromise timely and informed decision making by practitioners. As a result several recommendations were made and enacted by NHS trusts in terms of storage and organisation of content (Audit Commission, 1999). At a similar time there was concern about the ways in which service user information was being used and shared and how confidentiality was maintained, especially with increasing use of computer-held and shared records. In 1997, the Caldicott committee undertook a review of the use of patient information and the resulting report provided six general principles for good practice for patient-identifiable information, used within the NHS and local authority social care settings today. These principles are:

1. The information gathered and kept justifies the purpose.
2. The patient-identifiable information is absolutely necessary.
3. The minimum amount of identifiable data is kept as necessary.
4. Access to this information is on a need-to-know basis.
5. Those with access are aware and comply with their responsibilities.
6. Those with access understand and comply with the appropriate legislation.

The Caldicott report (DOH, 1997) also stipulated that each NHS trust and local authority had to appoint a nominated senior employee (known as Caldicott Guardians) to agree, review and monitor the systems in place for record keeping and use of service user data.

Health and social care professionals need to be continually aware of the wide range of legislation that impacts on service delivery and the keeping of care records. Therefore, in the UK the Department of Health have started an initiative alongside clinical and research governance, known as Information Governance (NHS Connecting for Health, 2007). This acknowledges that health and social care employees need adequate training to meet standards and best practice that comply with legislation, guidelines and professional codes of conduct (DOH, 2007b). A few of the most relevant pieces of legislation appertaining to the UK are discussed here.

The Public Records Act of 1958 identified that any record made or kept within any public service within the UK, including the NHS and the local authorities are public property, with each public service complying with the Act to ensure safekeeping, storage and eventual destruction of their records. Even though care records of deceased service users are considered public records, the Access to Health Records Act (1990) allows the executors or representatives of the deceased access to their health records. Sharing of information between practitioners working with children and young people has been made possible under the Children Act (2004).

The Data Protection Act (1998) considers the sharing, processing, access and type of information collected, stored and used about an individual (including photographic and audio media). On the other hand the Freedom of Information Act (1998) considers the sharing of information about the functioning of an organisation, to ensure transparency of information deemed to be in the public interest. The Data Protection Act (1998) also states that consent from an individual (whether service user or employee) is necessary to share that information with others. However there are some exceptions to this, especially when it is not in the public interest to obtain or rely on consent; that is in cases of notifiable infectious diseases, detection or prevention of crime or the protection of another individual (for example, a child). The Data Protection Act (1998) also complements the Human Rights Act (1998), which considers an individual's respect for privacy and family life, unless there is a legal requirement for disclosure.

Two relevant codes of practice that have been produced for NHS employees have been informed by the legislation already discussed, and also by the Caldicott report (1997) and the Audit Commission report (1999). These relate to confidentiality (DOH, 2003) and records management (DOH, 2006), which reiterate the need for confidentiality, best practice and security in the keeping of service user information as well as its management, storage and disposal.

Shared and integrated care records

The identified need and demand for records that are shared and integrated across and within organisations, and service users themselves has increased as part of person-centred care and practice. The recommendations made by the Climbié Inquiry (HMSO, 2003) and the UK government (Every Child Matters: Green Paper, 2003) for integrated working, plus the introduction of the single assessment process as part of Standard 2 of the National Service Framework for Older People (DOH, 2001) have reduced the duplication of assessment, documentation and information for children and older people in England and Wales.

Service users have reported that the duplication of assessment is poor use of time, which could be spent by professionals on the subsequent intervention or other issues (Ryan, 2005; DOH, 2006). The UK government has, therefore, extended the use of integrated working and documentation in its white paper *Our Health, Our Care, Our Say: A new direction for community services* (DOH, 2006). This identifies that by 2008 all adults with long-term health and social care needs can choose to have an integrated personal health and social care plan; this will be the norm by 2010.

Therapists have voiced concerns that the use of integrated records will 'dumb down' the specific needs of individual service users or specialist practitioners (such as allied health professions) in the desire for standardisation and consistency. Another issue raised is the possible medical focus on disease and impairment in health records rather than activity and participation (that is, functioning) (Thornquist, 2007). The need for well written, clear, concise documentation using agreed terminology is crucial within integrated documentation if records are shared or held by the service user. The challenge is to record information in a clear and logical way that avoids jargon and obscure abbreviations so that the documentation is readily accessible to both the service user and interprofessional team.

Increasingly, service users are holding their own health and social care records, as this is perceived to enhance transparency of information, empower users and enhance communication. In the UK and Canada, service users have a legal right to see their health and social care records. These user-held records (or patient-held records) are most commonly used in the community setting; people requiring home care or accessing maternity, mental health, cancer, diabetic and children's services. Even though this practice is increasingly commonplace, the efficacy of user-held records is currently uncertain (Jadad et al, 2003; Laugharne & Henderson, 2004).

Electronic care records

The increasing use of information and communication technology within health and social care has prompted international interest in the use of electronic care records (ECRs) that can be shared within and between organisations as well as with the individual service user themselves. The UK government has proposed that there will be unified electronic care records across statutory health and social care services by 2010 (Garner & Rugg, 2005). This has been driven by many of the policies already discussed and is a crucial part of both the single assessment process (DOH, 2001) and the Integrated Children's System (Every Child Matters, 2003). In many countries however, where there is no public health and social care system, the collaboration and sharing of electronic care records, though desirable, is potentially more problematic (Clarke & Meiris, 2006).

The potential of electronic records and service user data systems is that they allow efficient and faster booking of appointments, ordering repeat prescription medications, accessing records, communication with health professionals and provision of health information. The use of electronic care records will also be beneficial to service users as they will be able to access personal data more easily and, perhaps in the future, be able to identify who can access any part of their records (DOH, 2007c).

However, there is great concern about the security and confidentiality of such a national integrated system (Pagliari et al, 2007) and recent events in the UK have done nothing to dispel such anxiety amongst the public and health professionals alike (BMA News, 2008). Interestingly, Ryan (2005) expressed the opinion that instant electronic access to investigation results and updated records outweighs the need for confidentiality; many service users, such as those who are acutely ill, need pain relief or stress reduction as soon as possible. Ryan (2005) also suggests that paper records may be no more secure or reliable than electronic records that can be password protected, encrypted and audit trailed.

Allied health professionals in the UK have been strongly encouraged to participate in the design and implementation of electronic care records to ensure that these support and reflect professional practice as well as communicate the outcome of intervention (COT, 2007).

Content of documentation

The content of care records is crucial in providing the best possible care for service users. As already stated, good documentation should identify and allow for continuity of care across disciplines, organisations and also over time. The care records should be able to communicate factual information to the reader, clearly identifying the decisions made and the intervention, advice and services offered, and by whom. The treating therapist/health professional must be identified and the date and time of the intervention recorded. Documentary evidence of non-attendance, refusal of intervention, or repetitive or frequent intervention is also important.

Documentation needs to be clear and concise to ensure that no misunderstanding can occur. When writing reports, for example, it is necessary to consider who the 'audience' of the report will be when determining the content. As service users have the right of access to their records under the Data Protection Act (1998) therapists must ensure that records are documented in a clear and coherent manner to facilitate accessibility. As such, the therapist should be careful to use the appropriate clinical terminology and abbreviations.

Evidence of clinical reasoning and decision making should be demonstrated through the use of local protocols or therapy/care pathways, as well as through accurate recording of the assessment, intervention and evaluation process. To this purpose the use of problem-orientated medical records (POMRs) is a common feature within healthcare documentation throughout the world. POMRs were devised in the USA in the 1960s by Weed, establishing a scientific and systematic approach to documentation, which provided an accurate and comprehensive record of a service user's condition (Weed, 1968). POMRs are structured using the note keeping stages of 'SOAP':

■ subjective: service user's own story, usually in narrative form and in the service user's own words. Other history such as previous or co-existing medical conditions, family and social history would also be recorded here;

- objective: clinical observations and standardised assessment results;
- assessment: evaluation of situation from service user's history and the results of assessments and observations;
- plan: plan of intervention to address the issues raised; each of the issues raised in previous sections should be accounted for in this plan.

Although initially introduced as a paper-based system, Weed (1968) envisaged the POMR approach to be suitable for electronic/computerised systems. Originally designed for medical practitioners, the scheme has been readily accepted by many health disciplines throughout the world. However POMRs have been criticised for not communicating and recording the more qualitative, individual information from a service user's perspective (Chan & Spencer, 2005; Bossen, 2007) and have also been accused of being too cumbersome for use where a service user has complex health needs and/or has a prolonged period of care (Bossen, 2007).

The use of 'SMART' goals (specific, measurable, attainable, realistic and timely) is becoming increasingly common within care records to ensure that records are objective, relevant and logical in construction and explicitly demonstrate the therapist's clinical reasoning. The desire for objectivity and reduction in irrelevant documentation has lead to the drive for the use of standardised formats within record keeping. The use of nationally and internationally agreed minimum data sets has also been advocated, not only to collect data for statistical purposes but also to standardise the types of information that health and social care professionals are documenting. These data sets tend to be health condition specific and raise concerns that such a standardised format will not meet the needs of service users with either complex needs or multiple pathologies. In addition, they may be perceived as being entrenched with a medical model rather than a biopsychosocial model of care (McIntyre and Tempest, 2007).

The need for standardised terminology and coding of collected information is necessary, not only for clarity of recording, research and audit purposes but also for financial reimbursement of services provided by health and social care practitioners. For therapists working within publicly funded health and social care services the financial costs for their services to individual service users has not had great emphasis. However, the implementation of payment by results within the NHS will mean that healthcare providers will provide a service at a nationally agreed tariff. The need for greater transparency of the intervention carried out (for example, to provide value for money) will mean that therapists' activity will be coded; any therapy service activity left inaccurately or unrecorded will remain unpaid (Horton, 2007).

It is clear, therefore, that documentation of care records is an essential part of professional practice and not a low-priority activity. Therapists need to comply with, and understand, the principles of good practice, legislation, professional and local standards and guidelines. Therapists must be able to communicate clearly to colleagues and service users alike, explaining their clinical reasoning, risk management and decision making. They should be aware of not only with whom and how these records are shared and integrated, but also how to safeguard long-term continuity of care through accurate documentation. Other crucial aspects for consideration are that care records are also a means of collecting data for audit, research, service development and financial reimbursement. Good documentation ensures communication of our professional roles and identity.

The International Classification of Functioning, Disability and Health

Interprofessional and interagency working is dependent upon individual team members understanding their own roles as well as those of others. Productive teams are said to have clarity of their individual professional boundaries and at the same time have a mutual respect for the skills and abilities of other team members (Tempest and McIntyre, 2006). However, for a team of different professional and organisational backgrounds to work effectively, a common language and framework for practice is required to facilitate understanding and communication (Tempest and McIntyre, 2006). An appropriate model of practice needs to be chosen so that the beliefs and values of the team and individual team members are best met (Stamm et al, 2005). The International Classification of Functioning, Disability and Health (ICF) (WHO, 2001) has been advocated by many agencies as providing such a framework and common language for interprofessional working (Brintnell, 2002; COT, 2004; Intercollegiate Stroke Working 2004; NHS National Services Scotland, 2006; Sykes, 2007). This may be attributed to the fact that it was devised and has been validated by many professions and agencies worldwide, including the financial, legislative and governmental sectors as well as health and social care. The ICF is being increasingly used within allied health practice as a tool for research and practice. It is also used by service providers as a means of auditing allied health practice (NHS National Services Scotland, 2006).

The ICF is one of a family of classifications devised by the World Health Organization in 2001 to categorise the consequences of health conditions, and has global acceptance as a model of health and functioning by many professions, agencies and service users. Earlier attempts at classifying disability and providing a framework to communicate and understand disability, had a strong medical focus and were criticised by the International Disability Rights movement as not involving or listening to people with disability (Hurst, 2000). The ICF differs from previous models and classifications as it purports to be a bio-psycho-social model of health and functioning, considering health from a body, individual and societal perspective within an environmental context. The WHO devised this classification as a means to collect data on the *consequences* of health conditions across countries, services, disciplines and time, as well as to provide a common language to communicate effectively and reduce misunderstanding.

The ICF differs from other models of disability in that it is neutral, considering an individual and their health condition in terms of the interaction between their function and the context in which they live. Previous models, including the ICF's predecessor, the International Classification of Impairment, Disability and Handicap (ICIDH) (WHO, 1980) considered disability in a hierarchical way, with disability resulting from a health condition. However recent evidence demonstrates that many individuals feel disabled by society and their physical and attitudinal environment and not the health condition per se (Hurst, 2003).

How the ICF can be used

When establishing the service delivery, roles and activities of teams and its individual members, the ICF is a useful tool to establish the common issues for the client group and how these issues will be addressed and by whom. In Box 8.2, a client with multiple sclerosis is introduced and, in Figure 8.1, the key points are identified using the ICF framework.

The language and concepts within the classification have been used in Figure 8.1 to describe the issues for SA, and the appropriate codes have been added for the reader to consider the definitions of the concepts identified. By carrying out this exercise, teams can consider what

---

Box 8.2 SA, a lady with multiple sclerosis

SA was diagnosed 10 years ago with MS. Now aged 45, she is married with three children aged 20, 16 and 12. Her husband works abroad for most of the year as a freelance consultant engineer and their relationship is not close. All three children are living at home with the two younger children at the local secondary school. She worked as an actress until 3 years ago, losing her last contract because she was thought to be drunk. Her hobbies were watercolour painting and piano playing.

SA has recently deteriorated rapidly, requiring a wheelchair, and help with transfers and dressing. She is unable to do the housework or any domestic tasks. She is currently suffering from spasticity in both legs, tremor in her upper limbs, incontinence of urine and visual problems, as well as slurred speech.

SA feels depressed and isolated, as some friends are embarrassed by her current state. Her marriage is under strain as she feels she does not get much support from her husband. She feels a prisoner in her own home and is restricted to a ground floor room and bathroom only in their architecturally designed home, with her kitchen and living room accessible via one flight of stairs and the family bedrooms up a further two flights of stairs. Her children are her main carers and this is a great worry to her.

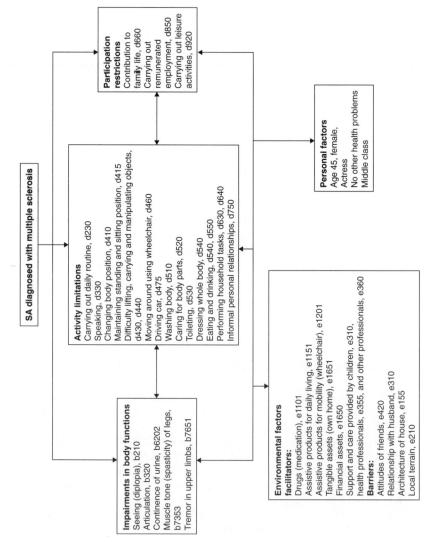

Figure 8.1 Using the ICF framework.

each team member is providing and what their intervention approach would be (for example, rehabilitative or compensatory). Where there are potential gaps or overlaps in provision, this can also be explored. For example an occupational therapist and physiotherapist may both want to consider wheelchair mobility (d465), however, the physiotherapist may want to address body function issues that help SA mobilise and transfer safely in the wheelchair (b7353, b7651) while the occupational therapist may be more involved in addressing SA's physical environment issues that may act as a barrier to independent mobility (e155, e210). By identifying which aspect of wheelchair mobility that the individual team members will address, the appropriate outcome measure can be chosen to evaluate the intervention for this activity limitation. Using the ICF as a framework for practice can facilitate team members to demonstrate their clinical reasoning and decision making, thus making team goals and interventions more transparent to the service user, carers and other involved agencies.

The use of the classification and the ICF framework has been documented within the literature where healthcare teams have compiled checklists and profiles specific to the needs of their clients with complex or chronic health conditions, listing the most appropriate domains and categories within the ICF components of body functions and structures, activity, participation and contextual factors (Rentsch et al, 2003; Steiner et al, 2002; COT, 2004). These authors describe how each team member took the lead and responsibility (with some overlap) of specific domains for assessment and intervention, linking the ICF domains with appropriate and compatible outcome measures. The authors described how team practice changed from discipline-specific verbal and written reporting and documentation, to ICF domain-specific reporting and documentation that was shared and integrated within the team (Rentsch et al, 2003; Steiner et al, 2003). Other services have utilised the ICF as a means of standardising and enhancing the quality of their care record documentation and have benefited from greater articulation of their clinical reasoning skills and professional profile within their teams (COT, 2004; Appleby and Tempest, 2006). The use of the ICF is also advantageous when considering electronic shared care records because of its international validation as a common language and framework, and the provision of codes for each item described. What is identified, however, is that training in the use of the ICF as a classification and framework is essential (Stucki et al, 2002; Rentsch et al, 2003; Appleby and Tempest, 2006; Verhoef et al, 2008) to ensure successful take-up of the ICF by interprofessional and inter-agency teams.

ICF core sets

The ICF, in its current form with approximately 1500 different categories, is considered to be too lengthy and unwieldy for everyday use.

Even though an ICF checklist has been devised, this too is considered lengthy and too generic in nature. As already discussed, clinical teams have already devised their own short lists of ICF domains and categories to assist their service in meeting the needs of their clients. The use of fewer more relevant ICF domains has been developed to produce several short lists known as core sets, suitable for use with specific health conditions or environments. Brief and comprehensive core sets have been developed involving focus groups of professionals and user groups; however not all core set development has involved users, carers or indeed allied health professionals (McIntyre and Tempest, 2007). Brief core sets have been developed for research purposes, while the comprehensive core sets are for practice (for example, the brief core set for stroke lists 18 categories and the comprehensive core set lists 130). It is hoped that in practice, the core sets enable teams to describe the issues for a client group, facilitate the outcome measure of choice and facilitate accurate documentation. Core sets are still undergoing validation around the world, and it is anticipated that their use will encourage teams to consider aspects and categories not traditionally examined (for example, contextual factors). However, there are some concerns that core sets will lead to less focus on an individual's functioning, with emphasis of examination of body functions and structures; moving away from a bio-psycho-social model of health and disability and back to a more medical model. Other concerns are that by 'pigeon-holing' clients by using core sets, it may be difficult to consider the needs of clients with multiple health conditions. Equally, core sets may facilitate a hierarchical focus on the health condition and its consequences rather than the dynamic interaction of the individuals' context and their health, which conflicts with current public health policy, stifling clinical reasoning, while encouraging prescriptive practice (McIntyre and Tempest, 2007).

The ICF is being increasingly used in everyday allied health professional practice, in the form of core sets for assisting service delivery, informing choice of intervention and outcome measures, and also in structuring care records and as a tool for audit, research and education. Although this classification is still undergoing development, allied health professions are supportive of its use in professional practice worldwide (Brintnell, 2002; Sykes, 2007).

References

Appleby, H., Tempest, S. (2006) Using change management theory to implement the International Classification of Functioning, Disability and Health (ICF) in clinical practice. *British Journal of Occupational Therapy* **69**(10), 477–480.

Audit Commission (1999) *Setting the Records Straight: A Review of Progress in Health Records Services*. London: Audit Commission.

BMA News (2008) The database that nobody wants? *BMA News* (February 2), 13.

Bossen, C. (2007) Evaluation of computerised problem-orientated medical record in a hospital department: does it support daily clinical practice? *International Journal of Medical Informatics* **76**(8), 592–600.

Brintnell, S. (2002) WHO – International classification of Functioning, Disability and Health – development and Canadian content. *WFOT Bulletin* **45**(5), 33–37.

Chan, J., Spencer, J. (2005) Contrasting perspectives following hand injury. *Journal of Hand Therapy* **18**(4), 429–436.

Chartered Society of Physiotherapy (2005) *Service Standards of Physiotherapy Practice*. London: CSP.

Clarke, J.L., Meiris, D.C. (2006) Electronic personal health records come of age. *American Journal of Medical Quality* **21**(3 suppl), 5S–15S.

College of Occupational Therapists (2004) *Guidance on the use of The International Classification of Functioning, Disability and Health (ICF) and the Ottawa Charter for health promotion in occupational therapy services*. London: College of Occupational Therapists.

College of Occupational Therapists (2006) *Guidance on Record Keeping*. London: College of Occupational Therapists.

College of Occupational Therapists (2007) *Electronic Care Records: Involving OTs in Design and Implementation*. London: COT.

Cumming, S., Fitzpatrick, E., McAuliffe, D., McKain, S., Martin, C., Tonge, A. (2001) Raising the Titanic: rescuing social work documentation from the sea of ethical risk. *Australian Social Work* **60**(2), 239–257.

Department of Health (1997) *Report on the Review of Patient-Identifiable Information*. Caldicott Report. London: Department of Health.

Department of Health (2001) *National Service Framework for Older People*. London: Department of Health.

Department of Health (2003) *Confidentiality: NHS Code of Practice*. London: Department of Health.

Department of Health (2005) *Confidentiality: NHS Code of Practice – Consultation*. London: Department of Health.

Department of Health (2006) *Records Management: NHS Code of Practice*. London: Department of Health.

Department of Health (2007a) *Independence, Choice and Risk: a Guide to Best Practice in Supported Decision Making*. London: Department of Health.

Department of Health (2007b) *NHS Information Governance: Guidance on Legal and Professional Obligations*. London: Department of Health.

Department of Health (2007c) *The Care Record Guarantee: Our guarantee for NHS Care Records in England*. London: Department of Health.

Every Child Matters (2003) *Integrated Children's Systems. London: Every Child matters.* http://www.everychildmatters.gov.uk/socialcare/integratedchildrensystem (Accessed 10th February 2008).

Garner, R., Rugg, S. (2005) Electronic Care Records: an update on the Garner Project. *British Journal of Occupational Therapy* **68**(3), 131–134.

Health Professions Council (2007) *Fitness to Practice Annual Report 2007*. London: HPC.

Her Majesty's Stationery Office (2003) *The Victoria Climbié Inquiry: Report of an Inquiry by Lord Laming*. http://www.victoria-climbie-inquiry.org.uk/finreport/6recommend. htm (Accessed 11th December 2007).

Horton, A. (2007) Payment by results: implications for occupational therapy practice. *British Journal of Occupational Therapy*, **70**(2), 85–87.

Hurst, R. (2000) To revise or not to revise? *Disability and Society*, **15**(7), 1083–1087.

Hurst, R. (2003) The International Disability Rights Movement and the ICF. *Disability and Rehabilitation* **25**(11/12), 572–576.

Intercollegiate Stroke Working Party (2004) *National Clinical Guidelines for Stroke*, 2nd edn. Clinical Effectiveness and Evaluation Unit. London: Royal College of Physicians.

Jadad, A.R., Rizo, C.A., Murray, M.W. (2003) I am a good patient, believe it or not. *British Medical Journal* **326**, 1293–1295.

Laugharne, R., Henderson, C. (2004) Medical records: patient held records in mental health. *Psychiatric Bulletin* **28**, 51–52.

McIntyre, A., Tempest, S. (2007) Two steps forward and one step back? A commentary on the disease-specific core sets of the International Classification of Functioning, Disability and Health (ICF). *Disability and Rehabilitation* **29**(18), 1475–1479.

NHS Connecting for Health (2007) *What you should know about Information Governance*. London: NHS Connecting for Health.

NHS National Services Scotland (2006) *AHPs Count: Developing Clinical data to inform the service about the work of AHPs*. ISD Scotland Publications. http://www.isdscotland.org/isd/servlet/FileBuffer?namedFile=AHPs_Do_Count.pdf&pContentDispositionType=inline (Accessed 28th March 2008).

Nursing and Midwifery Council (2007) *Record Keeping Guidance*. London: NMC.

Pagliari, C., Detmer, D., Singleton, P. (2007) Potential of electronic personal health records. *British Medical Journal* **335**, 330–333.

Rentsch, H.P., Bucher, P., Dommen, Nyffler I., et al. (2003) The implementation of the International Classification of Functioning, Disability and Health (ICF) in daily practice of neurorehabilitation: an interdisciplinary project at the Kantonsspital of Lucerne, Switzerland. *Disability and Rehabilitation* **25**(8), 411–421.

Ryan, T.E. (2005) A patient's perspective on medical records. *Artificial Intelligence in Medicine* **36**, 119–120.

Stamm, T.A., Cieza, A., Machold, K., Smole, J.S., Stucki, G. (2005) Exploration of the link between conceptual occupational therapy models and the International Classification of Functioning, Disablity and Health. *Australian Occupational Therapy Journal* **53**(1), 9–17.

Steiner, W.A., Ryser, L., Huber, E., Uebelhart, D., Aeschlimann, A., Stucki, G. (2002) Use of the ICF as a clinical problem-solving tool in physical therapy and rehabilitation medicine. *Physical Therapy* **82**(11), 1098–1107.

Stucki, G., Ewert, T., Cieza, A. (2002) Value and application of the ICF in rehabilitation medicine. *Disability and Rehabilitation* **24**(17), 932–938.

Sykes, C. (2007) *WCPT Keynotes: Health Classifications 2 – Using the ICF in clinical practice*. http://www.wcpt.org/common/docs/keynotes/ICF2.pdf (Accessed 10th January 2008).

Tempest, S., McIntyre, A. (2006) Using the ICF to clarify team roles and demonstrate clinical reasoning in stroke rehabilitation. *Disability and Rehabilitation* **28**(10), 663–667.

Thornquist, E. (2007) Patient records – physiotherapists' contributions. *Advances in Physiotherapy*. iFirst Articles 1–10 (Accessed 12th December 2007).

Verhoef, J., Toussaint, P.J., Putter, H., Zwetsloot-Schonk, J.H.M., Vliet Vlieland, T.P.M. (2008) The impact of introducing an ICF-based rehabilitation tool on staff satisfaction with multidisciplinary team care in rheumatology: an exploratory study. *Clinical Rehabilitation* **22**(1), 23–27.

Weed, L.L. (1968) Medical records that guide and teach. *New England Journal of Medicine* **278**(11), 593–600.

Wood, D.L. (2001) Documentation guidelines: evolution, future direction and compliance. *The American Journal of Medicine* **110**(4), 332–334.

World Health Organization (1980) *International Classification of Impairment, Disability and Handicap*. Geneva: World Health Organization.

World Health Organization (2001) *International Classification of Functioning, Disability and Health*. Geneva: World Health Organization.

9: Preparation for professional practice: evidence-based practice

Sally Spencer

Evidence-based practice is not about *doing* research, it is about finding, appraising and using the best available research in daily practice. The most well known and frequently used definition of evidence-based practice is from Sackett et al (2000:1) as follows, 'the integration of best research evidence with clinical expertise and patient values'.

The most important feature of this statement is that it advocates an integrative approach to healthcare, involving both the clinical professional and the patient in the decision-making process. It is a commonly observed fallacy, particularly among students, that the evidence-based healthcare movement seeks to remove the professional, and the patient, from the business of care. On the contrary, without the healthcare professional and the patient, the fundamental building blocks of evidence-based healthcare, namely the body of evidence on a given topic, could not exist. Healthcare professionals conduct and patients take part in evaluations of interventions that form the foundations of the evidence base.

The term 'evidence' is important here and can be conveniently described as follows, 'reliable observational, inferential, or experimental information forming part of the grounds for upholding or rejecting claims or beliefs' (Hurwitz, 2004:1024). In short, it is an accumulated set of information conforming to an acknowledged set of quality standards – a body of good quality research studies.

So why is evidence-based practice so important? The easiest way to answer that question is to look at the alternative: practice that is not based on evidence. This approach would instead use personal knowledge and experience, information from colleagues, and perhaps information from locally available research publications.

One of the problems with this approach lies in the volume of information. When healthcare was in its infancy little was known about effective treatments and practice was largely based on experimentation with individual patients to find a solution that worked. However, advances in healthcare kept pace with developing communication networks, and knowledge of effective treatments were initially passed by word of mouth, then through professional institutions and their associated publications. The volume of information on healthcare treatments is now so unimaginably vast that no single individual can retain all of it. Instead, modern practitioners rely on libraries and other information repositories to collate this material so that it can be easily accessed. So, relying purely on your own local experience would exclude potentially vital information from other practitioners and researchers in the global environment.

A second problem is bias. A non-evidence-based approach relies on the knowledge and experience of the individual, which is naturally subject to personal preference and prejudices, some of which will not be evidence based. A simple example might be that a therapist decides to treat all future cases of acute lower back pain with prolonged bed rest because they recently successfully treated a patient using this approach. The decision to generalise this treatment fails to acknowledge the limitations of the evidence, e.g. success may have been due to specific characteristics of the individual, the patient may not have actually taken the bed rest, and so on. Most importantly of all, *the patient may have recovered spontaneously without the intervention*. In the absence of a formal research study there is no means of attributing causality to the recovery. There is also no indication, from the single and apparently positive observation, whether the intervention may be harmful for other patients.

The non-evidence-based approach is wrong for a whole host of reasons and ethically indefensible if good evidence is available to suggest that alternatives are preferable. When the outcome of treatment is harmful in some way, the non-evidence-based approach strays into the realms of professional negligence if a treatment regimen was pursued contrary to the evidence. In a world where patients are better informed about standards of care, litigation in healthcare is becoming increasingly common. One commentator on the relationship between evidence and medical negligence has suggested that 'increasingly, it will be possible to plead just one particular form of negligence: failing to follow guideline X' (Hurwitz, 2004:1025). Given that so many professional practice guidelines are based on evidence, it is yet another reason to ensure that practice is evidence based.

Several professional institutions have issued standards that reflect the need for practitioners to stay abreast of the best evidence in their field and to ensure it features in day-to-day practice. This is not only in line with the recent evidence-based healthcare movement, and current government policy, but it also ensures that the professions evolve and develop practices consistent with high-quality research into the best care for patients.

The Professional Standards for Occupational Therapy Practice (College of Occuaptional Therapists, 2007:4) include intervention and evaluation standard statements. This is an explicit requirement that interventions should be selected on the basis of evidence. The 'Service quality and governance standard statements' include standards 1 and 3 respectively as follows:

▪ Occupational therapists should maintain and develop their knowledge, skills and behaviour, and therefore their competence to practice.
▪ Occupational therapists should provide a service of consistent quality, in line with local, professional and national standards.

These standards carry an implicit assumption that practitioners should maintain practices that are underpinned by the best available evidence. The maintenance of knowledge implies the updating of healthcare information in line with evidence-based developments in research, many of which are manifest in treatment guidelines and national service frameworks.

Similarly the Service Standards of Physiotherapy Practice (Chartered Society of Physiotherapists, 2005) incorporate Service standard 4:

- There is a system to ensure that all physiotherapists provide care that is based on the best available evidence of effectiveness.

This standard specifies criteria that include provision of evidence-based information resources and training that enable practitioners to use, evaluate and implement research evidence.

We have established that evidence-based practice is important for the welfare of both practitioners and patients, and that it is a feature of professional standards. We should now consider in more detail what constitutes high-quality evidence in the context of treatment interventions.

What constitutes good evidence?

The 'gold standard' method for evaluating whether an intervention works in the healthcare setting is unequivocally the randomised controlled trial (RCT). In a recent article in the Journal of the American Medical Association, Califf (2005:489) suggests,

> . . . a trial of adequate size to show modest but important effects on true clinical outcomes must remain the standard for the evidence on which therapies are based.

However, it is not the ideal method for answering all questions about healthcare. For example, you cannot use an RCT to evaluate interventions where harm is the expected outcome, such as looking at smoking in relation to lung cancer, because of the ethical issues relating to the prospective allocation of participants to the smoking arm of a trial. (See McKee (1999) for a discussion of the merits of non-randomised trials where randomisation procedures are not possible.) If you wanted to know about patients' views on a particular aspect of service, a survey or qualitative research using focus groups may be more appropriate than an RCT.

So, an RCT is the best method for evaluating appropriate interventions. Why? What is so special about an RCT? The main aim of any study evaluating an intervention is to find out whether it works, to establish efficacy. In order to do this you need a study design that will be as fair as possible and the strength of the RCT design lies in the principle of the fair test. It is the responsibility of study investigators to authentically test whether the intervention works and this can be achieved in a number of ways: by comparing it to a group not receiving the intervention, to demonstrate that it is better than nothing at all; by comparing it to a group receiving a carefully matched placebo intervention, to demonstrate that it has genuine efficacy; or by comparing it to a group receiving standard care or an alternative, to test it against current practices.

RCTs commonly incorporate several of these elements in a single design in order to answer several questions at once. For example, Pfleger et al (1992) investigated the efficacy of various forms of chest physiotherapy for patients with cystic fibrosis. The study had five arms and was designed to answer several questions. A control group was used to determine whether physiotherapy was better than nothing, in this case 'nothing' was defined as spontaneous coughing. This was compared to two new physiotherapy techniques. The positive expiratory pressure mask (PEP) was the first intervention and autogenic drainage (AD) was the second intervention. In addition, in order to compare these single interventions with a combination therapy and to control for effects in the order that therapies were delivered, the study included PEP followed by AD as the third intervention and AD followed by PEP as the fourth intervention. A fifth intervention could have been introduced here comparing the above groups with physiotherapy given as standard practice. However it could be argued that it made more sense to do this as a follow-on study in order to keep the design relatively simple.

The components of an RCT are designed to allow those questions to be answered under controlled conditions to ensure the test is as fair as possible, and that means eliminating bias from the design, conduct and analysis of the study. It is not the purpose of this chapter to describe the RCT design. Readers are directed toward a series of statistical notes and articles published in the British Medical Journal (Roberts & Torgerson, 1998; Altman & Bland, 1999; Torgerson & Roberts, 1999; Day & Altman, 2000; Altman & Schulz, 2001).

Empirical research from several studies provides fairly compelling evidence that lack of randomisation, poor randomisation procedures and lack of blinding can result in inflated estimates of treatment effects, i.e. biased results (Schulz et al, 1995; Kunz & Oxman, 1998; Gluud, 2006). So, although the RCT design is the ideal for evaluating the effects of interventions, the quality of individual studies is variable and practitioners need to be able to critically evaluate studies in order to assess quality, which in turn will influence interpretation of the study findings. On the issue of bias in clinical trials, Gluud (2006:493) has noted that, 'appraising bias control in individual trials is necessary to avoid making incorrect conclusions about intervention effects'.

Where do I find the evidence?

At this point you are probably feeling rather deflated at the prospect of having to critically appraise research studies that are often highly complex and difficult to understand. The good news is that much of this work has been done for you. The National Institute for Health and Clinical Excellence (NICE) is a National Health Service organisation responsible for providing guidance on promoting good health and preventing and treating ill health in England and Wales (http://www.nice.org.uk/). Scotland has a similar organisation, the Scottish Intercollegiate Guidelines Network (SIGN) (http://www.sign.ac.uk/). The two organisations differ in their inclusion of cost-effectiveness factors in the appraisal of evidence. Preference for one system over another is a matter of debate, not about the value of economic factors per se, but whether they should influence guideline recommendations. My own view is that evidence of effectiveness should be the primary concern and that cost-effectiveness and cost-implication issues should be managed at the level of the consumer. This allows for variation in local needs and economic climate to set agendas and to prioritise the uptake of evidence. The process of producing guidelines involves collating evidence that meets a set of quality criteria, and producing recommendations for treatment and practice based on that evidence. NICE guidelines and appraisals are distributed to key members of primary care trusts (PCTs) and hospitals throughout the UK to ensure that the guidelines reach relevant practitioners within the organisation. NICE grades the evidence by design and conduct of the study. A summary of the NICE hierarchy of evidence is shown in Table 9.1.

You may be surprised to note that RCTs are not at the top of this table. Systematic reviews of RCTs are considered the best level of evidence.

Table 9.1 National Institute for Health and Clinical Excellence (NICE) – levels of evidence.

Ia	High-quality meta-analyses, systematic reviews of RCTs, or RCTs with a very low risk of bias
Ib	Well conducted meta-analyses, systematic reviews of RCTs, or RCTs with a low risk of bias
Ic	Meta-analyses, systematic reviews of RCTs, or RCTs with a high risk of bias
IIa	High-quality systematic reviews of case-control studies. High quality case-control or cohort studies with a very low risk of confounding, bias or chance and a high probability that the relationship is causal
IIb	Well conducted case-control or cohort studies with a low risk of confounding, bias or chance and a moderate probability that the relationship is causal
IIc	Case-control or cohort studies with a high risk of confounding, bias or chance and a significant risk that the relationship is not causal
III	Non-analytic studies (for example, case reports, case series)
IV	Expert opinion, formal consensus

That is because a single RCT, even if it is well designed and executed, may not adequately reflect the whole of the population being studied. For example a single trial of occupational therapy for Parkinson's disease may have included predominately men, or women, or a limited age range. The trial may be limited in other ways, such as the sample size or its range of health outcomes, and therefore insufficient as the basis for global treatment recommendations.

In order to be as certain as possible of the efficacy of a given treatment, all of the evidence from similar trials should be combined together. This process of evidence synthesis is a systematic review and may differ in important respects to a conventional literature review. The aim of a systematic review of the effectiveness of an intervention is to collate *all* the relevant trials on a given question. The aim is to provide a fair and balanced summary of the effectiveness of the intervention and, where feasible, to provide clarity on such issues as side effects. For example, we might consider in a systematic review the evidence from RCTs evaluating occupational therapy for Parkinson's disease. This synthesis of the accumulated data may involve the statistical combination of results from different studies in a meta-analysis, or where that is not possible because the studies are too different, a narrative combination of the study findings. Where there are conflicting results, the review can clarify the overall picture, make recommendations for practice and highlight areas where new research is required. For these reasons, among others, well conducted systematic reviews are considered the top of the evidence tree.

NICE was set up in 1999 and SIGN in 1993. The business of evaluating evidence and producing guidelines can be a lengthy process and consequently there is a limited number of completed guidelines and appraisals. However, NICE and SIGN are not the only organisations to evaluate evidence of efficacy. There is a robust information infrastructure to support practitioners in their search for and use of appropriate evidence and much of this is freely available through the Worldwide Web. A table at the end of the book lists a selection of these resources.

Systematic reviews represent the best evidence on the effects of interventions. However, the quality of reviews varies widely, from unsystematic reviews, where the evidence is limited by factors such as databases searched or language and year of publication, to rigorously conducted reviews where evidence is collated using a formal framework. The Cochrane Collaboration publishes systematic reviews on the Cochrane Library that empirical evidence has shown 'are more rigorous and better reported than those published in peer reviewed journals' (Jadad et al, 2000:537). This methodological rigour means that Cochrane reviews are the acknowledged 'gold' standard for systematic reviews. The Collaboration has been in existence since 1993 and is divided into 51 Cochrane Review Groups, each of which concentrates on a specific area of healthcare.

Reviews are completed by people from a variety of backgrounds in healthcare and largely without remuneration. The current edition of the Cochrane Library contains 3298 systematic reviews and 1755 protocols, which are design templates for forthcoming reviews. The Library also contains 15 Fields that draw together healthcare issues impacting on many review groups. The Cochrane Rehabilitation and Related Therapies Field was instrumental in the creation of the physiotherapy database PEDRO and the occupational therapy database OTseeker and is now part of the Centre for Evidence-Based Physiotherapy, all of which are listed at the end of this book.

One of the great strengths of Cochrane Reviews, and one of the ways in which they differ from most other reviews, is that they are updated. Where most reviews are produced as a finite exercise in evidence collation and therefore out of date as soon as new research becomes available, Cochrane Reviews are revised when new evidence, in the form of new high-quality research, becomes available. So, as an evidence resource it occupies a unique position as an evolving database. Needless to say, Cochrane Reviews are routinely included as high-quality evidence in guidance published by organisations such as NICE and SIGN.

The 2007 edition of the Cochrane Library includes reviews of therapies, for example, 'Chest physiotherapy for preventing morbidity in babies being extubated from mechanical ventilation', by a group of Australian reviewers for the Cochrane Neonatal Group (McLauchan & Handoll, 2001). Of the completed reviews published on the Cochrane Library, 94 reviews include interventions within the physiotherapy domain. These reviews are from 20 Cochrane Review Groups and 36% of the reviews were produced by reviewers in the UK. The earliest review was published in 1998 and there is an upward trend in the number of physiotherapy reviews published annually, with 21 published in 2007.

The library also includes, 'Occupational therapy for rheumatoid arthritis' by a group of Dutch reviewers for the Cochrane Musculoskeletal Group (Steultjens et al, 2004). Of the reviews published on the Library, ten reviews include interventions that fall into the occupational therapy domain. These reviews are from six Cochrane Review Groups and seven were produced by UK reviewers. The earliest review was published in 1998 (Robertson et al, 1998) with sporadic publications in the intervening period and three published in 2007 (Dixon et al, 2007; French et al, 2007; Hoare et al, 2007).

A large percentage of these 104 therapies reviews show inconclusive results and recommend further research. In many cases clear conclusions were limited by the quality of the trials. Problems range from no trials that meet the review entry criteria, to trials with poor randomisation procedures. There is a need for good quality efficacy trials across the healthcare spectrum for physiotherapy and especially for occupational therapy, where there is only a handful of reviews.

How to evaluate the evidence

The dearth of good quality evidence brings us back to the issue of evaluating the evidence that *is* available. The evidence base comprises a range of materials, including controlled trials, RCTs, reviews of effects and practice guidelines. Some resources, such as PEDRO and Cochrane, provide quality rating criteria for the material they review but it is essentially up to practitioners to evaluate evidence quality. There are several freely available tools that can help with this critical appraisal process.

The Critical Appraisal Skills Programme (CASP) (http://www.phru. nhs.uk/casp/casp.htm) produced by the Public Health Research Unit of the NHS in the UK includes critical appraisal checklists that can be downloaded (for systematic reviews, RCTs, cohort studies, qualitative research). The checklists are relatively simple to follow and enable practitioners to evaluate study quality in a standardised manner. Tools and resources are also available at the Centre for Evidence Based Physiotherapy, Occupational Therapy Evidence Based Practice Research Group, OTseeker and PEDRO. For evaluating practice guidelines the Appraisal of Guidelines Research and Evaluation (AGREE)(19) tool has been approved by both NICE and SIGN and is available at the following website: http://www.agreecollaboration.org/.

Implementing evidence-based practice

The availability of good-quality evidence is no guarantee that it will change practice. Even when a body of evidence is used to develop guidelines, their influence on day-to-day practice is not necessarily guaranteed. Research by Hyman and Pavlik (2000) showed that many physicians based hypertension therapies on blood pressure thresholds above those recommended in national guidelines and that much of this was attributable to lack of awareness of the guideline recommendations. However, a survey of UK general practitioners indicated that the use of evidence-based information did influence day-to-day practice (Tovey and Godlee, 2004).

Several authors have suggested that the influence of guidelines on practice is dependent on a range of factors. A review by Grimshaw and Russell (1993) suggests that guidelines can change practice if introduced within a rigorous development, dissemination and implementation structure. Similar results were reported in a more recent review of the uptake of NICE guidance, which showed that, although there was variability in implementation across the healthcare spectrum, it was most successful in organisations where a framework existed for supporting the implementation of guidance (Sheldon et al, 2004). This framework included professional support, a convincing evidence base and organisational systems for tracking the implementation of guidance.

The specific nature of the implementation effort also appears to influence the likelihood of changing practice. Recent research by Lockwood et al (2004) showed that a system of regularly scheduled evidence-based meetings in one UK institution ensured that treatments were more closely aligned with published evidence. Underpinning the variability in evidence uptake is a growing body of research showing that improved knowledge does not always result in behaviour change. A review by Coomarasamy and Khan (2004) showed that teaching alone improved knowledge of evidence-based methods and practices but did not change actual practice behaviour. The most effective method of changing behaviour was through the integration of evidence-based teaching with clinical practice. This largely involved the development of an appropriate question and search strategies, appraisal of evidence and application of findings within the context of current clinical problems or cases. However, Strauss and Jones (2004) have pointed out that more research is required on the impact of evidence on practice behaviours in order to focus efforts in the right areas to ensure that evidence is realised in practice.

Glasziou and Haynes (2005) have proposed an evidence 'pipeline' or framework for getting evidence into practice that incorporates both practitioner and patient issues. It includes raising awareness and acceptance of evidence, ensuring that knowledge and infrastructure are available to support change, and gaining patient agreement and adherence to change. For practitioners seeking to implement evidence-based practice, this 'pipeline' provides a framework to ensure evidence translates into practice.

In summary, the implementation of evidence is most likely to be successful if there is organisational/institutional support and monitoring, and if dissemination and teaching for practitioners are set in the context of current practice.

What to do if there is little evidence on interventions currently in use

Following a comprehensive search of available resources you may find little evidence. This can take several forms.

Firstly, you may find that there are almost no studies that have evaluated the intervention that you are interested in. A commonly used tenet under these circumstances is that *absence of evidence is not evidence of absence*, in other words just because you can't find evidence that it works doesn't mean that it doesn't work. It means that proof of efficacy is still to be acquired and the acquisition of that proof will involve the conduct of good quality RCTs. There is an additional important point to make with regard to absence of evidence and that relates to safety. Absence of evidence might be misconstrued as suggesting there is *no* evidence of harm, but just because there is no *evidence* of harm doesn't mean we should infer that the intervention is free from harm. In this instance, proof from studies evaluating negative as well as positive effects of interventions are still required.

Secondly, you may find that there are no good quality studies, insufficient studies or conflicting studies that render interpretation difficult. In this case further research studies are required to clarify the uncertainty. Help with these problems can be found at the James Lind Alliance which endeavours to prioritise treatment uncertainties by involving both patients and clinicians (http://www.lindalliance.org/).

Thirdly, you may find that evidence exists, in the form of a number of clinical trials, but that a synthesis of these studies does not exist. An overview of the studies may be required in order to inform a wide range of local practices and/or to resolve conflicting results. This situation requires a systematic review of the available evidence. Practitioners wishing to undertake a review are advised to contact an appropriate Cochrane Review Group with a proposed title for a systematic review. The Collaboration may provide free training and support to assist in the development of a systematic review.

In summary, in the absence of evidence for the effectiveness of interventions currently in use, it is advisable to establish proofs through the conduct of high-quality clinical trials. However, that recommendation is on the proviso that there is *no* evidence of harm.

References

Altman, D.G., Bland, J.M. (1999) Statistics notes: how to randomise. *British Medical Journal* **319**, 703–704.

Altman, D.G., Schulz, K.F. (2001). Statistics notes: concealing treatment allocation in randomised trials. *British Medical Journal* **323**, 446–447.

Califf, R. (2005) Simple principles of clinical trials remain powerful. *Journal of the American Medical Association* **293**(4), 489–491.

College of Occuational Therapists (2007) *Professional Standards for Occupational Therapy Practice*. London: College of Occupational Therapists.

Chartered Society of Physiotherapy (2005) *Service Standards of Physiotherapy Practice*. London: The Chartered Society of Physiotherapy.

Cluzeau, F.A., Littlejohns, P., Grimshaw, J.M., Feder, G., Moran, S.E. (1999) Development and application of a generic methodology to assess the quality of clinical guidelines. *International Journal for Quality in Health Care* **11**(1), 21–28.

Coomarasamy, A., Khan, K.S. (2004) What is the evidence that postgraduate teaching in evidence based medicine changes anything? A systematic review. *British Medical Journal* **329**, 1017–1021.

Day, S.J., Altman, D.G. (2000) Statistics notes: blinding in clinical trials and other studies. *British Medical Journal* **321**, 504.

Dixon, D., Duncan, D., Johnson, P., Kirkby, L., O'Connell, H., Taylor, H., Deane, K.H.O. (2007) Occupational therapy for patients with Parkinsons disease. *Cochrane Database of Systematic Reviews* 2007, Issue 3. Art. No.: CD002813.

French, B., Thomas, L.H., Leathley, M.J., Sutton, C.J., McAdam, J., Forster, A., Langhorne, P., Price, C.I.M., Walker, A., Watkins, C.L. (2007) Repetitive task training for improving functional ability after stroke. *Cochrane Database of Systematic Reviews* 2007, Issue 4. Art. No.: CD006073.

Glasziou, P., Haynes, B. (2005) The paths from research to improved health outcomes. *Evidence Based Medicine* **8**(2), 38–38.

Gluud, L.L. (2006) Bias in clinical intervention research. *American Journal of Epidemiology* **163**(6), 493–501.

Grimshaw, J.M., Russell, I.T. (1993) Effect of clinical guidelines on medical practice: a systematic review of rigorous evaluations. *Lancet* **342**, 1317–1322.

Hoare, B.J., Wasiak, J., Imms, C., Carey, L. (2007) Constraint-induced movement therapy in the treatment of the upper limb in children with hemiplegic cerebral palsy. *Cochrane Database of Systematic Reviews* 2007, Issue 2. Art. No.: CD004149.

Hurwitz, B. (2004) How does evidence based guidance influence determinations of medical negligence. *British Medical Journal* **329**, 1024–1028.

Hyman, D.J., Pavlik, V.N. (2000) Self-reported hypertension treatment practices among primary care physicians. Blood pressure thresholds, drug choices, and the role of guidelines and evidence-based medicine. *Archives of Internal Medicine* **160**(15), 2281–2286.

Jadad, A.R., Moher, M., Browman, G.P., Booker, L., Sigouin, C. (2000) Systematic reviews and meta-analyses on treatment of asthma: critical evaluation. *British Medical Journal* **320**, 537–540.

Kunz, R., Oxman, A.D. (1998) The unpredictability paradox: review of empirical comparisons of randomised and non-randomised clinical trials. *British Medical Journal* **317**, 1185–1190.

Lockwood, D., Armstrong, M., Grant, A. (2004) Integrating evidence based medicine into routine clinical practice: seven years' experience at the Hospital for Tropical Diseases, London. *British Medical Journal* **329**, 1020–1023.

McLauchlan, G.J., Handoll, H.H.G. (2001) Interventions for treating acute and chronic Achilles tendinitis. Cochrane Database of Systematic Reviews. 2; CD000232.

McKee, M., Britton, A., Black, N., McPherson, K., Sanderson, C., Bain, C. (1999) Methods in health services research: Interpreting the evidence: choosing between randomised and non-randomised studies. *British Medical Journal* **319**, 312–315.

National Institute for Health and Clinical Excellence (April 2007) *The Guidelines Manual*. London: National Institute for Health and Clinical Excellence. Available from: www.nice.org.uk.

Pfleger, A., Theissl, B., Oberwaldner, B., Zach, M.S. (1992) Self-administered chest physiotherapy in cystic fibrosis: a comparative study of high pressure PEP and autogenic drainage. *Lung* **170**(6), 323–330.

Roberts, C., Torgerson, D. (1998) Understanding controlled trials: randomisation methods in controlled trials. *British Medical Journal* **317**, 1301–1310.

Robertson, L., Connaughton, J., Nicol, M. (1998) Life skills programmes for chronic mental illness. *Cochrane Database of Systematic Reviews* , Issue 3. Art. No.: CD000381.

Sackett, D., Strauss, S.E., Richardson, W.S., Rosenberg, W., Haynes, R.B. (2000) *Evidence-Based Medicine – How to Practice and Teach EBM*, 2nd edn. London: Churchill-Livingstone.

Schulz, K.F., Chalmers, I., Hayes, R.J., Altman, D.G. (1995) Empirical evidence of bias. Dimensions of methodological quality associated with estimates of treatment effects in controlled trials. *Journal of the American Medical Association* **273**(5), 408–412.

Sheldon, T.A., Cullum, N., Dawson, D., Lankshear, A., Lowson, K., Watt, I., et al. (2004) What's the evidence the NICE guidance has been implemented? Results from a national evaluation using time series analysis, audit of patients' notes, and interviews. *British Medical Journal* **329**, 999–1006.

Steultjens, E.M.J., Dekker, J., Bouter, L.M., van Schaardenburg, D., van Kuyk, M.A.H., van den Ende, C.H.M. (2004) Occupational therapy for rheumatoid arthritis. Cochrane Database of Systematic Reviews.1; CD003114.

Strauss, S.E., Jones, G. (2004) What has evidence-based medicine done for us? *British Medical Journal* **329**, 987–988.

Torgerson, D., Roberts, C. (1999) Understanding controlled trials: randomisation methods: concealment. *British Medical Journal* **319**, 375–376.

Tovey, D., Godlee, F. (2004) General practitioners say that evidence based information is changing practice. *British Medical Journal* **329**, 1043.

10: The golden thread of continuing professional development – continuing professional development and professional portfolios

Margaret Gallagher

This chapter discusses the mandatory continuing professional development (CPD) requirements of the Health Professions Council and explores a variety of approaches in order to guide newly graduated practitioners and returning professionals to meet the standards while integrating CPD into their professional practice.

The need for a more rigorous approach to the regulation of health and social care professionals was the most significant outcome of service failures such as the Bristol Royal Infirmary Inquiry (2001). Public accountability and the ability of the professional to ensure and promote current competence are integral to this new framework. CPD is now a mandatory requirement for all healthcare professionals but within a framework where the individual practitioner is both self-directed and autonomous. The aim of CPD is to demonstrate the current competence of the healthcare professional, and provide evidence of this competence through a portfolio which satisfies the need for public accountability.

When contemplating your individual CPD it is wise to reflect on the broad context in which you will be practising and consider who the stakeholders in the process are. The stakeholders include the individual professional, the professional bodies (Chartered Society of Physiotherapists, and the British Association of Occupational Therapists), the regulators (Health Professions Council) and the public. For this process to work, enabling the graduate professional to become a lifelong learner, the goals of CPD have to be meaningful and have inherent integrity for the individual. The approach which is chosen to identify CPD needs is an important part of the process and helps to ensure a successful outcome. The use of reflective practice, clinical supervision and mentoring should contribute to the development of the CPD plan. Clinical governance in healthcare is one of the quality assurance processes which aim to support clinical competence and manage risk more effectively (Department of Health, 1998).

For occupational therapists and physiotherapists the Health Professions Council (HPC), as the statutory regulator, sets the framework through which CPD will be audited from 2008. The professional bodies, the British Association of Occupational Therapists and the Chartered Society of Physiotherapists (CSP), also provide guidance so that the practitioner can meet the requirements within the context of their practice environment. CPD is a lifelong process of self-directed activity (College of Occupational Therapists, 2002), which should be voluntary, described by Alsop (2000:19) as 'a professional responsibility and as a process for maintaining competence in practice'.

The time required for CPD is frequently a contentious point, whether it should be the individual practitioner's time or the organisation's (employer's) time. A joint position statement by the ten health professional bodies and two royal colleges of nursing provides explicit guidelines on the amount of time that they regard should be protected as necessary for a professional to maintain their competencies, excluding mandatory training (Royal College of Nursing, 2007). They recommend 6 days (45 hours) of protected time to undertake CPD annually. The HPC has no power to force employers to provide time for CPD, but clearly encourages them to support best practice. CPD is costly in organisational and individual terms, both in time and financial resources and should therefore be planned and carefully monitored during an individual's career progression.

There are numerous approaches to CPD, including significant technological innovations such as the CSP (2008) development of a web-based approach to maintaining CPD. Practitioners should consider a variety of options that can meet their CPD needs.

What is continuing professional development

In 'The New NHS: A first class service: quality in the new NHS', the Department of Health (1998:43) described CPD as,

> a process of life long learning for all individuals and teams that meets the needs of patients and delivers health outcomes and health priorities of the NHS that enables professionals to expand and fulfil their potential.

This indicates the broad societal importance of CPD within the NHS. More specifically the NHS in Scotland (2003) used the Madden and Mitchell definition (1993:12) to guide the discussions relating to CPD as,

> the maintenance of and enhancement of knowledge, expertise and competence of professionals throughout their careers according to a plan formulated with regard to the needs of the professional, the employer, the profession and society.

The HPC's definition also includes reference to safe practice, recognises the potential for the evolving scope of practice (HPC, 2006) and encourages the concept of lifelong learning. However there is no consensus on what constitutes CPD (Griscti & Jacono, 2006).

The terms CPD and continuing professional education (CPE) are frequently used interchangeably, with for example the Canadian Association of Occupational Therapists using the term CPE, which embraces a comprehensive notion of progressive professional development including both formal and informal learning opportunities (CAOT, 2006).

There is an interesting point of contention relating to CPD activities as a mandatory requirement of regulators and professional bodies, and a possible conflict with adult learning theory, which identifies the individual's motivation as the key element in adult learning theory (Pearson, 1998). This potential conflict is highlighted by Magill-Cuerden (2007), where CPD that is identified by the professional may be at odds with that which is mandatory and imposed by management. Another consideration is that the stress of undertaking continuing professional education needs to be recognised and suggests that planned long-term CPD with targeted resources is a more appropriate way for organisations to manage the process. The final suggestion is that sharing the responsibility across all levels within the organisation would have the aim of empowering individual members of staff (Magill-Cuerden, 2007).

An important factor in relation to improving the performance of healthcare services, identified by Ham (2003), was to recognise the motivation of healthcare staff, which is to offer a high standard of service. Strategies that appeal to this motivation, such as professional education and development, are more likely to be successful than tighter regulation. This indicates that a focus on the education and training of clinicians to achieve a new balance between the highly valued autonomy and public accountability would produce better services (Ham, 2003). Research undertaken with nurses in Ireland (Joyce & Cowman, 2007), indicates that the key issue for successful CPD is the individual's motivation for engagement in postgraduate education. This suggests that there are important implications for resource allocation for CPD and raises the question of how motivation is taken into account when allocating CPD resources (Joyce & Cowman, 2007). Given the importance of the individual's motivation and their professional autonomy, the challenge that managers have to address is to balance the needs of the organisation with those of individual professionals within the organisation (Kennerley, 1992).

In a study with community-based physiotherapists, Bourne et al (2007) found that the requirement to be evidence-based practitioners is not necessarily supported in practice, as they had difficulty in accessing resources to research practice. They also found that the majority of the participants had no CPD objectives, and where practitioners had such objectives they felt more positive about the process and their usefulness.

The important question of what impact CPD has on practice was explored in a small study by Tennant and Field (2004) with intensive therapy unit nurses, where the focus was on the evaluation of the CPD. They found that the course did have an impact on practice, and in addition nurses on the unit who did not attend the course also developed their practice. This raises interesting questions about the sharing of good practice and knowledge which is a key factor in adult learning.

The effective use of reflection in supporting a professional learning culture is an important component of professional development and is highlighted in a study considering professionalism in medical education (see Chapter 3).

A review of the literature in nursing has indicated that the effectiveness of CPD remains unexplored (Griscti & Jacono, 2006), also making the point that there is an element of preaching to the converted, as motivated competent staff did engage in CPD activities. Some key themes emerged from this review, such as, for CPD to be effective the learning methods need to be participatory, and that a needs analysis should be undertaken. The question of including the service user in the evaluation of the effectiveness of CPD is also raised (Griscti & Jacono, 2006). It has proved difficult to demonstrate the link between the cost effectiveness of CPD and healthcare outcomes as the research has been very limited (Brown et al, 2007). Resource allocation for CPD, both in time and financial resources, will be of concern to everyone involved in undertaking or delivering CPD.

When reviewing your CPD it may be useful to consider the term 'advanced practitioner' which has been defined by Alsop (2003:262) as that which:

> will make additional demands that will take you beyond the realm of merely remaining competent in a changing world. It will demand energy and commitment to developing your potential to a different level.

Given the demands of professional practice this may be a helpful concept to explore within the context of professional progression and CPD.

Context of CPD

The Department of Health (UK) has made explicit the link between continued competence and the quality of patient care (Department of Health, 1998, 2004). Developments in medical technologies and practice present a bewildering challenge at times, requiring healthcare professionals to be positively engaged in maintaining the currency of their practice and continually developing their skills. There have also been changes in public expectations of health and social care, which has been reflected in Department of Health policies such as the Expert Patient (Department of Health, 2001) and the Commission of Patient and Public Involvement in Health (2007). These policies express the requirement for healthcare and social care professionals to design and deliver services with the service user as a partner in the process. These twin requirements of maintaining competencies and integrating the service user's perspective into professional practice are key drivers within the current context of practice.

The Knowledge and Skills Framework (KSF) (Department of Health, 2004) also aims to support the development of individual professionals which is linked to an assessment of competencies. Within this framework the process of preceptorship for new graduates has been designed to support their integration into the service setting, including an assessment of their competency and pay progression. In a study in Ireland (Joyce & Cowman, 2007), the most important factor in nurses undertaking post-registration education was the possibility of promotion (see Chapter 12). A study of clinical nurse managers indicates that providing CPD opportunities may be an important factor in enhancing job satisfaction (Gould et al, 2001) and therefore could be a vital link in the recruitment and retention of skilled, motivated professionals.

What are the current HPC requirements?

The HPC standards (HPC, 2006:8) state that registrants must:

1. Maintain a continuous, up-to-date and accurate record of their CPD activities.
2. Demonstrate that their CPD activities are a mixture of learning activities relevant to current or future practice.
3. Seek to ensure that their CPD has contributed to the quality of their practice and service delivery.
4. Seek to ensure that their CPD benefits the service user.
5. Present a written profile containing evidence of their CPD upon request.

(See HPC web site for further suggestions for CPD activities: www. hpc-uk.org.)

Ways of ensuring you meet the requirements

We know from research that the motivation of the individual is important when undertaking CPD (Magill-Cuerden, 2007) and that it should be a voluntary (Alsop, 2003) participatory activity (Griscti & Jacono, 2006). Organisational commitment is necessary at all levels, and appealing to professional's motivation to provide high-quality services through CPD opportunities may deliver better patient outcomes than introducing additional regulation (Ham, 2003). Health care professionals value access to appropriate learning resources, not only to keep their practice current but also to meet identified CPD objectives (Bourne et al, 2007). CPD can have an impact on practice, but evaluation of the CPD activities needs to be integrated into the process (Tennant and Field, 2004). We also know that finding time for CPD is not easy but understanding what assists and where the potential barriers are may help in developing an effective approach to CPD.

The HPC describe five categories of CPD activities: work-based learning, professional activity, formal education, self-directed, and other activities. This sets a very broad canvas for CPD which can include the more obvious professionally focused activities, but also includes duties or roles that are performed outside the professional role such as community volunteering.

For the new graduate the approach adopted for CPD and developing a portfolio will inevitably be influenced by the context of your first post. This will depend on the demands of the service, the supervision and management received, and the aspirations individuals have for the future. From the individual perspective the most important factor is to have a clear idea of the shape of your future career. Knowing what you want, for example if you want to work with children, will help you plan your career objectives.

Benefits of CPD

The best way to look at the benefits that CPD and portfolio development offer to the novice practitioner is to view this as a self-directed approach to career progression. Taking ownership of the process may empower you to evaluate where you have been, where you are now, and think where you want to be in the future. This approach will assist the maintenance of your career and competencies over time and through service changes, with the aims of reducing the risk of individuals dropping out of the profession and maintaining their interest and commitment for the profession.

The scenarios in Boxes 10.1 and 10.2 outline the real world challenges newly qualified therapists need to overcome when considering their future careers. Have you devised your own career pathway? Read the two scenarios below. Consider how the therapists could approach their CPD more effectively.

Box 10.1 Scenarios and real world challenges

I am a band 5 physiotherapist currently working in an acute trust inpatient service, and have rotated through musculo-skeletal, neurological, medical and respiratory specialities. Mandatory training is provided, and I attend the band 5 development programme. My long-term plan is to specialise in working with neurological patients. While working on the neurological ward I have discussed my interest in neurology with the senior neuro-physiotherapist who provided clinical teaching through double treatment sessions with patients. I belong to ACPIN, the neurological clinical interest group of the CSP, and have attended a conference for which I paid, and this has enabled me to develop my network of professionals in this speciality. CPD and portfolio development is encouraged within the trust, but I find I have to undertake these activities in my own time. Supervision happens when I request it.

Box 10.2 Scenarios and real world challenges

I am a band 5 occupational therapist working within a service for people with learning disabilities. I have just finished my preceptorship year. I feel that my first year of practice has been about increasing my understanding of my responsibilities to ensure I am developing and evidencing my practice. The trust supports CPD and as a new graduate I enrolled on a band 5 development programme. I was given a portfolio to evidence my development over the course of the year and this counted towards fulfilling the dimensions within the KSF and standards of practice for the HPC. I undertook mandatory and internal training within the trust on a continual basis. The trust is also implementing a new way of delivering the OT process and staff are invited to attend fortnightly training sessions. This is also considered as CPD. Supervision has been important to me but has not been as frequent or of a quality that I had hoped for, so I have sought informal and formal support from additional sources. I expected that part of my role would be to research evidence-based examples of good practice to ensure I was working effectively. I had also hoped that CPD time would be provided for me to explore avenues of enquiry and development that matched my professional interests and aspirations. However in fulfilling the requirements of my trust and the HPC, I have had little time to engage in activities autonomously which would support my future career.

General advice

- **Plan**: try to be focused about where you would like to be in 2–5 years time. For example if you aim to be a consultant therapist, your profile will require an MSc and research experience. If you know what speciality you want to practise in be clear and share this with your line manager and/or supervisor.
- **Think broadly**: opportunities for CPD are not just located in structured, formal work-based environments. Explore the community for volunteering opportunities which can align with your career objective, for example volunteering through charities such as SCOPE, Headway or Mencap to gain more experience of working with the client group you are interested in.
- **Supervision**: clinical supervision can be a very effective contribution to CPD. The 'just right' challenge within a supervisory relationship should be beneficial in the development of clinical reasoning and professional development. However this relies on the relationship working well, which is not always the case. There are structured training programmes offered by NHS trusts to improve the quality of supervision in practice, and it is advisable to engage in this important conversation.
- **Reflective practice**: the effective use of reflective practice will support your professional development; for further guidance please see Chapter 3.

- **Professional bodies**: become a member of your professional association, and be an active member. Being engaged in the activities of your association will provide you with experience and responsibilities, while offering a very valuable network of contacts which maybe of assistance in the future. Start by supporting the association, either locally or nationally, by attending meetings. Offering to take the minutes of meetings or assisting with the administration of a specialist section is an excellent way of understanding the role of the association and what your contribution may be. Within the associations there are also specialist sections, which are the groups that develop and facilitate good practice guidelines that are so important in delivering evidence-based practice.
- **Mentor**: you may need a mentor to help guide you to your career objectives. A programme described by Wilding et al (2003), MentorLink, has been created to assist practitioners in ongoing professional development. Initially developed for occupational therapists, it is now being joined by other health professionals. While a structured programme such as MentorLink has proved helpful, informal mentoring relationships with senior members of your profession can be a positive aspect of the healthcare domain, and should be encouraged.
- **CPD is not limited by the HPC standards**: CPD offers you the option of both integrating the HPC standards and transcending them. Consider them a useful baseline for your career progression, as a framework to position yourself appropriately for the next phase in your career.
- **Creativity:** just because CPD and a professional portfolio are mandatory requirements, do not exclude creativity and imagination. The important point to remember is that CPD includes a vast range of activities which may be useful in developing professionally.
- **Peer review**: find out from colleagues who are prepared to share their approach to CPD, how they have developed their CPD and portfolio. This is a practical way of establishing how others are conceptualising their CPD and portfolio, and the discussion may help to initiate some ideas of your own, which you can share with them.
- **Annual performance reviews**: given the link between annual reviews and pay progression as required by the KSF (Department of Health, 2004), there is a potentially difficult line between identifying individual strengths and areas for development. Approaching the process with honesty will assist you and the line manager to identify appropriate resources and experiences that will contribute to CPD. The key outcomes from the review are the objectives, including professional development, which provide a baseline from which evaluation can take place.
- **Evaluation**: as a part of the reflective process, routine critical evaluation of the effectiveness of the CPD plan will help establish if you are on course for the desired career direction.
- **Who pays?** This is a vexed and contentious issue due to the cost constraints within health and social care. Professionals are expected to

take ownership of their CPD, which may require individuals taking responsibility for paying in part or fully for postgraduate education and training that is not mandatory.

■ **Practice/clinical educator**: consider the role of a practice educator as contributing to your CPD profile. The role is critical for the future of the professions, and most universities offer training and support for this.

■ **Research**: this may initially appear forbidding, but as a graduate you will be equipped to start to engage in the research process through the pre-registration programme. You can contribute in various ways to research projects, by supporting colleagues and developing your research interests through specialist sections, for example.

Making CPD work for you: the portfolio

As with most professional activities there is guidance about what is good or best practice. For new graduates, developing a portfolio can be considered as a beneficial professional habit, and the sooner that this is integrated into your view of practice the more effective this will be. The purpose of a portfolio should be to deliver documentary evidence of personal and professional progression:

> A portfolio helps professionals define and track professional and personal goals.
>
> (Nagayda et al, 2005:7)

This highlights the importance of both having objectives and their regular review.

Alsop (2000:9) suggests conceptualising the portfolio into your past, present and future professional activities, describing a portfolio as:

> dynamic in that it needs to be updated to reflect ongoing needs and opportunities.

It is important to consider the confidentiality of a portfolio as you may use the whole or part to demonstrate competence or fitness for a particular purpose. This may require the selective use of elements of a portfolio to fit a particular purpose, remembering that this is your personal portfolio.

A good place to start a portfolio is with your curriculum vitae (CV), as this provides an opportunity to reflect on relevant aspects of past experiences (see Chapter 11). Reviewing your current practice and professional role enables you to take stock of your position, particularly in relation to agreed objectives. The critical evaluation of the current situation will help with refining current and future career objectives. Identifying a career path for the short (1 year), medium (2–3 years) and long term (3 years plus) will give a clear focus to the process. This will assist the plan for the future, as you will consider what course of action is needed to achieve these objectives.

This North American approach includes the potential use of a portfolio in not only demonstrating current competence but also as a business tool. A development of this is the pitch book, which is described as a selective summary of a particular aspect of your practice and development for a particular purpose, such as a selection panel or a business opportunity (Nagayda et al, 2005). Given the expanding range of employment opportunities in the statutory, voluntary and independent sectors, a pitch book maybe a useful way to prepare for such events.

Nagayda et al (2005) suggest that the level of experience the professional has influences and determines the approach to the development of a portfolio, describing categories as entry-level, intermediate, advanced, re-entry (as in returning to practice) and indirect or non-traditional roles. This approach has the merit of helping to focus on the particular developmental and changing needs of the practitioner as they progress in their career.

The design and development of your portfolio may be driven by, and the content determined by, the regulatory requirements from the HPC. However there is room for imagination and creativity in how this is expressed within the portfolio. Be mindful that a portfolio is a live document which will change as your career develops, and consequently requires regular revisions. Including patient and service user feedback can be a very constructive approach to demonstrating their involvement in your career and service development.

Undertaking CPD and developing your portfolio can assist your metamorphosis from the undergraduate to the graduate professional who is able to demonstrate their current competencies and areas that will need further development. As part of this metamorphosis you may have to shed ideas and approaches which you once held to be appropriate, but in the light of research and experience are now no longer effective. Consider CPD as the golden thread which both challenges and unites your career. Positive engagement in CPD will enable professional and personal growth, and may also sustain you through the more demanding aspects of practice. CPD may also help you develop your own artistry as a healthcare professional within the science of practice.

References

Alsop, A. (2000) *Continuing Professional Development: a Guide for Therapists*, 3rd edn. London: Blackwell Science.

Alsop, A. (2003) The leading edge of competence: developing your potential for advanced practice. In: G. Brown, S. Esdaile, S. Ryan (eds) *Becoming an Advanced Healthcare Practitioner*. London: Butterworth Heinemann.

Bourne, J., Dziedzic, K., Morris, S.J., Jones, P., Sim, J. (2007) Survey of the perceived professional, educational and personal needs of physiotherapists in primary care and community settings. *Health and Social Care in the Community* **15**(3), 231–237

Bristol Royal Infirmary Inquiry (2001) *Public Involvement Through Empowerment*, Chapter 28 www.bristol-inquiry.org.uk/ (Accessed 28th October 2007).

Brown, C.A., Belfield, C.R., Field, S.J. (2007) Cost effectiveness of continuing professional development in health care: a critical review of the evidence. *British Medical Journal* **324**, 652–655.

Canadian Association of Occupational Therapists (2006) *CAOT Position Statement. Continuing Professional Education.* www.caot.ca/default.asp?ChangeID=163&pageID= 153 (Accessed 2nd November 2007).

Chartered Society of Physiotherapists (2008) *Eportfolio system pilot* www.csp.org.uk/director/ newsandevents/physioalerts.cfm?item_id=457DF3E2BD30A6DF90EAE6EBAE0BA081 (Accessed 1st January 2008).

College of Occupational Therapists (2002) Position Statement on Lifelong Learning. *British Association of Occupational Therapy* **65**(5), 201–206.

Commission for Patient and Public Involvement in Health (2007) *Annual Report 2006/7.* London: The Stationery Office.

Department of Health (1998) A *First Class Service: Quality in the New NHS.* London: Department of Health.

Department of Health (2001) *The Expert Patient: A New Approach to Chronic Disease Management.* London: The Stationery Office.

Department of Health (2004) *The NHS Knowledge and Skills Framework (NHS KSF) and the Developmental Review Process, final version.* London: Department of Health.

Gould, D., Kelly, D., Goldstone, L., Maidwell, A. (2001) The changing training needs of clinical nurse managers: exploring issues for continuing professional development. *Journal of Advanced Nursing* **34**(1), 7–17.

Griscti, O., Jacono, J. (2006) Effectiveness of continuing education programmes in nursing: literature review. *Journal of Advanced Nursing* **55**(4), 449–456.

Ham, C. (2003) Improving the performance of health services: the role of clinical leadership. *The Lancet* **361**, 1978–1980.

Health Professions Council (2006) *Your Guide to our Standards for Continuing Professional Development.* London: HPC Park House. Available at www.hpc-uk.org.

Joyce, P., Cowman, S. (2007) Continuing professional development: investment or expectation? *Journal of Nursing Management* **15**(6), 626–633.

Kennerley, J.A. (1992) Managing professionals and professional autonomy. *Higher Education Quarterly* **46**(2), 166–173.

Madden, C.A., Mitchell, V.A. (1993) *Professions Standards Competence: a Survey of Continuing Education for the professions.* Bristol: University of Bristol.

Magill-Cuerden, J. (2007) Leading and managing professional development – improving patient care. *Journal of Nursing Management* **15**(6), 563–566.

Nagayda, J., Schindehhette, S., Richardson, J. (2005) *The Professional Portfolio in Occupational Therapy: Career Development and Continuing Competence*. New Jersey: Slack Inc.

NHS Education for Scotland (2003) *Making Continuing Professional Development Work*. Edinburgh, Scotland: NHS.

Pearson, A. (1998) The competent nurse and continuing education: Is there a relationship between the two? *International Journal of Nursing Practice* **4**, 143.

Royal College of Nursing (2007) *A Joint Position Statement on Continuing Professional Development for Health and Social Care Professionals*. London: Royal College of Nursing.

Tennant, S., Field, R. (2004) Continuing professional development: does it make a difference? *British Association of Critical Care Nurses, Nursing in Critical care*, **9**(4), 167–172.

Wilding, C., Marais-Strydom, E., Teo, N. (2003) MentorLink: empowering occupational therapists through mentoring. *Australian Occupational Therapy Journal* **50**(4), 259–261.

11: Preparation for health and social care employment

Mandy Jones and Judith McIntyre

Introduction

Historically, healthcare professionals have held an envied position within the job market, with the number of vacant posts far outweighing the number of applicants. This has allowed new graduates the luxury of almost being able to 'pick' the city, and possibly the institution, where they would like to apply for work. However, more recently the situation has completely reversed (see Chapter 12). This change in circumstances has led to intense competition for graduate employment, together with the realisation that effective self-marketing is essential in order to secure a junior post.

This chapter aims to explore the changes affecting health and social care employment, and identify possible strategies which may be used by graduates to make the transition into their first post.

Changes to health and social care sector

The marked change in public sector employment has occurred secondary to changes in service delivery within health and social care. The changes aimed to deliver comprehensive care in line with other international care organisations, while retaining the distinctive National Health Service (NHS) structure, which is open to international scrutiny (Iliffe & Munroe, 2000; Lewis & Gilliam, 2001). Over the past few years, the implementation of these structural changes has begun to impact on the recruitment processes and, therefore, on the transition of students into what used to be assured employment as newly qualified health and social care professionals.

The NHS reforms have not been made in isolation; they reflect global changes that have striven to make professionals produce more work of a higher quality. This has been epitomised by the implementation of new clinical governance standards to exercise greater managerial control over clinical activities, so that clinical excellence may flourish (Lewis & Gilliam, 2001). This change dictates more emphasis on clinical professionals to work within an evidence-based practice approach that integrates individual clinical expertise with the best available external clinical evidence from systematic research. The focus is now on the effectiveness of the healthcare system, concentrating as much on 'value for money' as on any other quality outcome (Iliffe & Munroe, 2000).

Accordingly, health and social care students must focus on both the academic and the practical sides of their higher education courses. However, students must also learn to sell not just the training aspect of their studies to an employer but also themselves as a brand that reflects their tone and manner, and therefore the values and unique personality that will allow them to fit into an employing organisation.

To change behaviour so that more focus is placed on developing the employability skills of students on their courses is possible; but such a change requires a more comprehensive approach than is generally being carried out on health and social care degree courses at present. This means that some time should be spent exploring the dynamics of the social and health care employment market and for courses to train and develop the relevant employability skills of these professionals to successfully compete in the recruitment market. In other words, it is not enough to just give students the practical and professional experience required to do their job. They need to get a first job in an ever changing and competitive employment market, which can only be done by encouraging students to explore further the world of work they will be entering and the potential employers' expectations of sector graduates.

The recruitment market – what changes?

Historical changes in the labour recruitment market have seen a shift away from the traditional industrial society to a more knowledge-led society. Within higher education, this phenomenon was recognised as occurring as early as the 1960s, when The Robbins Report on Higher Education (HMSO, 1963) suggested that higher education was not effectively preparing undergraduates for the world of work. This was followed in the 1970s by Prime Minister Jim Callaghan's Ruskin College speech (Callaghan, 1976), which heralded a drive to create an education–employer interface where the focus was on preparing students to meet the needs of industry. Callaghan argued that 'there are complaints from industry that new recruits do not have the basic tools to do the job' (ibid:3).

These changes in the economy have demanded a highly skilled labour force which is driven towards the pursuit of knowledge, and where the expansion in technology also requires that individuals have greater knowledge and skills related to information technology (IT). It is for this reason that the emphasis on the importance of skills development within higher education has increased, especially with respect to the role of universities in preparing all their students for future work and careers (UGC, 1984; White Paper, 1987).

Harvey and Green (1994) stated that despite these government changes, which were indeed essential to the relationship between work and higher education, a survey of employers' views at the time showed that they continued to be dissatisfied with the level of skills all graduates were displaying in employment. Harvey and Green (1994) drew on a survey conducted on 258 managers and recent graduates, which found that employers wanted adaptive, adaptable and transformable people to help them maintain, develop and transform their organisation in response to and in anticipation of change. In the light of this continued dissatisfaction regarding graduates entering employment, the skills debate was given more emphasis. The government set up an inquiry headed by Sir Ron Dearing (Leitch, 2005) to address these concerns.

The skills debate

Where the Dearing Committee (1997) highlighted the fact that changes in the economy were affecting the higher education curriculum, the Leitch report (2005), some years later, identified the need for the UK to identify its optimal skills to maximise economic growth, productivity and social health. However, they both recognised the need to improve skills so that innovation and growth may be driven forward. It was Dearing (1997), however, who focused on higher education and recognised the major part it needed to play in preparing undergraduates for the ever changing role of employment, identifying a 'plethora' of skills that existed within the curriculum.

With no one quite knowing what skills they were meant to be developing, four generic skills were proposed as 'key skills' (Dearing, 1997:17), which the committee considered universities should adopt in the higher education curriculum. These skills were communication, teamwork, problem solving and leadership. They were considered to be the core 'employability skills' that would be most relevant in the relationship between the higher education curriculum and employment. The concept was to embed employability skills programmes in the higher education curriculum, rather than provide them as bolted-on skills development programmes, although it was argued that these programmes would be seen as optional by members of the academic staff and students and would therefore be unlikely to attract undergraduates' full attendance.

Embedded skills within health and social care degree courses?

Currently, professional skills embedding within health and social care degree courses is delivered through interprofessional education. This forms a module that is delivered within the final year of the health and social care degree courses. The module is designed to inform students of new and innovative collaborative work procedures and processes within and between public sector organisations, drawing on relevant learning and practice skills development plus professional interaction. However, due to the vast extent and scope of this module, its focus on employability skills can only amount for a small fraction of the time available.

Yet a crucial element of interprofessional education is the emphasis it places on shared learning by two or more professions (Regan De Bere, 2003). This involves a genesis of new kinds of working and new kinds of professional roles, through novel combinations of tasks and responsibilities, which can be exchanged while competencies are developed. Additionally, the students I see on a regular basis have mentioned that the learning and skills development within interprofessional education are remote from the employability requirements they come across when looking for a job.

A study undertaken by Cooper and Spencer-Dawe (2006) on 198 first-year students from four interprofessional groups established that all the students involved in the programme found that working alongside other service users was beneficial; it gave them an awareness of the practical issues involved in working within a team and a realisation that in order to provide holistic care they need to work closer with service users. The students also identified the importance of interpersonal communication skills. They felt well equipped for one-to-one communication and networking, although they had all found that establishing and maintaining communication with other busy professionals called for persistence and was time consuming.

The students thought their individual personal attributes predisposed them to be natural communicators and networkers, but felt that, although they had gained the required skills and confidence in proportion to their life experience, this did not help them in successfully identifying the attributes required for employment (Barker et al, 2005).

The same study on interprofessional education for collaborative patient-centred practice (IECPCP) showed that 'champions', who help to persuade others to support specific interprofessional education programmes (Freeth et al, 2005), are key elements. It is through their role in implementing interprofessional education that communication with stakeholders and other agencies about professional requirements becomes more defined. Champions are often able to suggest where resources might be found to support the different interprofessional programmes and act as advocates for political and organisation changes that may affect the programmes.

Indeed, where evidence-based practice appraises research findings to support decisions about best practice, clinical effectiveness requires high-quality evidence-based guidance to ensure the provision of effective care. The skills new professionals gain in their jobs are always specific to the job and they do not realise their transferability within the employability circuit. The individual professional is not sufficiently embedding these generic core skills or demonstrating how they will effectively use them within the workplace.

Similarly, problem-based learning is a move towards a self-directed and flexible learning approach to help students close the gaps between what they are taught and what they encounter in practice in the work situation (Davys & Pope, 2006). It is hoped this will again close the gap between theory and practice and, at the same time, will be a pragmatic process that leads to employment.

Regan De Bere (2003) states that interprofessional learning has a positive approach, but evidence of the nature of impact on practice is less illuminating. 'Professional education alone does not equate to professional development' (ibid:105); as such it cannot be assumed that interprofessional education will always lead to improvements.

It seems as if interprofessional learning, therefore, is doing its job in that it is upholding the value of practice-based learning as an essential component in the preparation of working in the health and social care environment, where collaboration and partnership are essential to providing effective practice. However, it cannot be taken for granted that interprofessional education by its nature also prepares students for a seamless entry into employment.

Hammick (2000) insists that more research is needed on the effectiveness of learning within the interprofessional education programme. Research also needs to be undertaken into whether interprofessional practice is indeed providing graduates with the skills required for competing in the market for jobs in their specialist sector.

Encountering the workplace

Within the employment recruitment process, demonstrating the acquisition of specific skills and their transferability within the workplace setting and in the context of the employers' recruitment expectations from candidates, is critical. Nybø (2004) proposes that job advertisements now reflect the changing workplace setting of a competency-based approach. This takes the focus away from the traditional job-based human resource practices and replaces it with competence-based value-creating processes that determine the individual's ability to be adaptive, adaptable and transformative.

As such, graduates will need to demonstrate their ability to fit into the organisation's culture, be willing to learn and add to knowledge and skills, and use these attributes in the face of change. They will need to interact effectively as well as analyse, critique, synthesise and enable leaderships as well as look ahead (Harvey et al, 1997). An individual will, therefore, be recruited according to the knowledge and skills required by the workplace. Because the individual competencies need to match the complexity of workplace tasks, the knowledge and skills will have to be of a standard that allows the individual to work effectively and innovatively, and to be an expert within their given field (Nybø, 2004). Although skills and knowledge are standardised within the social care sector through intensive training, which makes behaviour predictable and less arbitrary, students still have to be distinctive in their approach to potential recruiters.

This new world of health and social care sector employment, referred to as 'the third way' by Tony Blair (Barr, 2000), is based on partnership and driven by performance. This means that newly qualified health and social care professionals are finding the recruitment process challenging in more ways than one. Indeed, at one British university, the destination statistics of health and social care workers, collected 6 months after graduation, shows that since 2003/2004, newly qualified professionals who responded to the annual higher education statistics agency (HESA) government survey are finding it increasingly difficult to enter employment upon graduation. The percentage of newly qualified health and social care professionals entering the profession directly after graduation fell to 79% in 2005/2006, a decrease of 12 percentage points, compared to 91% in 2003/2004 (Brunel University, 2004).

This trend demonstrates that changes to the employment sector are directly affecting the career prospects of newly qualified professionals. They do not all appear to enter employment, up to 6 months after graduation; this was the tradition until 5 years ago.

This paradigm is somewhat synonymous with the assertion of Bate et al (2004) that there is an international realisation and understanding that the design of the existing health care system will not deliver what is required for the future. An approach is therefore required that will allow learners to adopt strategies that will permit them to develop more effective methods to contribute to their all-round learning (D'eon, 2005).

One such built-in strategy involves the raising of awareness of the realities of the workplace through a more holistic, interactive style of teaching so that they can freely realise their own attributes and strengths, seek to develop their weaknesses, and sing their own praises in order to greet the changing employment environment with confidence. This may also create a greater determination to succeed and a better emphasis on learning and skills transferability into the wider world (Jarvis, 2006).

Eraut (1994) refers to the personal and propositional knowledge of a person, which he states is easy to separate when describing a student's learning, skills and experiences. However, when it comes to effectively marketing themselves as professional practitioners, Eraut (ibid) points out that they will also be required to demonstrate both personal and propositional knowledge. It is the synergy between the two forms that demonstrates the specific processes of learning, development and its prospective professional application. And it is this which will make for a successful applicant entering the health and social care sector.

Health and social care students are often enthusiastic about how a clinical placement provides them with first-hand experience of their chosen career. They also describe how it allows them to develop the skill of interacting with others in a workplace setting, helping them to understand the social processes that are taking place and to interpret the activities and interactions that take place. From this standpoint, it is clear that new health and social care professionals now have to take stock of their experiences, apply attention to detail and confer a meaning to the evidence of their practice on placement. They cannot take their learning, knowledge, or skills for granted but must allow their emergent identity to be interpreted and taken into consideration by the employer (Holmes, 2000).

These interpretations help to predict the future performance of the graduate, so that a judgement on the degree of skills and competences learnt at university can be made. This judgement will then determine whether the employer feels able to recruit the graduate, and if they do so, to anticipate the graduate's performance and progression over a period of time.

Competency-based recruitment

Of the students who come through my office door, many appear to be surprised by the emphasis placed by employers on a diverse range of abilities that do not always focus on their professional portfolio of competences. One NHS health and social care employer recently told me that 'we are now looking for a rounded individual' – this has to be reflected in both the application and at interview and must go beyond the applicant's specific knowledge and skills.

The emphasis on competency-based recruitment has now extended its tentacles from private industry to public employment organisations that allow for a more rigorous approach to recruitment. This provides an opportunity for the employer to predict the candidate's future behaviour in the workplace by ensuring clarity in statements and expressions, preventing personal bias and making sure that claims made by candidates are genuine.

Applicants will therefore need to demonstrate evidence of their energy, drive and ambition, ability to act as a team player, and that they possess enough confidence, initiative and creativity to make a difference to the organisation, its clients and other stakeholders. Employers will be looking at defining the role of the job within the different competencies they judge as required by the post-holder.

Perkins and Salomon (1994), in referring to interpersonal skills of graduates, state that students have to develop those skills in order to cope with the changing economic market. They suggest that where the traditional higher education curriculum has been remote in its delivery to the wider world context, much of what undergraduates are learning should also relate not only to the graduates' academic study and the promotion of client care, but also to how learning and performance in one setting prepare the student to learn the rules, habits and knowledge appropriate in another.

While these competency-based communication and interpersonal skills are being assessed within the health and social care sector, students often do not realise the importance of demonstrating them within the recruitment process. More competition is giving health and social care employers the opportunity to raise the stakes, and this is reflected in recruitment procedures. This is partly being manifested in the long interview process that new graduates are now experiencing when applying for jobs.

Duffy et al (2004) also mention the emphasis on communication and interpersonal skills. Within the health and social care sector, communication skills include obtaining a patient's medical history, giving therapeutic instructions and information needed for informed consent to undergo diagnosis and therapeutic procedures, providing counselling to motivate participation in therapy and its basis for writing objectives, and designing assessment measures. Interpersonal skills are relational and process orientated. This aptitude also focuses on the effect of communication on another person, and this includes respect for others, paying attention to verbal, non-verbal and intuitive communication channels, being personally present in the moment, mindful of the importance of relationships and having a caring intent, not only to relieve suffering but also to be curious about and interested in the clients' ideas, values and concerns.

Duffy et al (2004) also referred to clinical teamwork with peers, colleagues and myriad others. In the health and social care sector this means speaking up, providing clarity by ensuring ideas are precise and understood, demonstrating attentiveness to different roles and exchanging tasks and support processes within the team. Duffy et al (2004), however, revealed that communication and interpersonal competencies within health and social care teams are usually learned through a hidden curriculum of on-the job training, or not all. Because of the abstruse manner in which these attributes are learned, it can be generally assumed that not all students are enlightened as to how to transfer these skills or demonstrate their competencies, especially when it comes to effective self-marketing for employment. Certainly that is my experience from the students that I see.

Practice-based education and clinical placements are providing students with a holistic approach to their work. It is this which is meant to be standardising their skills, and creating social capital in terms of building self-confidence and self-belief (Hilton & Morris, 2001; Nybø, 2004). Ayas and Zenuick (2001) agree that within this system of learning in communities, opportunities are presented to all students – not only to develop their competencies on the job but also to be fit for purpose. This provides undergraduates with the scope to witness at first hand how industry and higher education work together so that information feedback occurs. They are also able to make choices that will provide them with a way forward towards realising further individual, academic and employment goals, plus skills transfer for those goals to be achieved.

All higher education courses present to some extent, an invisible, unexpressed expectation to students of what employers want from graduates, but these concealed expressions sometimes hide a mismatch between the core skills that universities are teaching and those that employers want from the graduating force. In referring to meta-skills, a process that can only be judged as having developed within the given employment context in which the skills are related, Holmes (2000) states that it is only through this process that entry to or performance within occupation areas can be facilitated or inhibited. This involves an awareness of skills learning and the acquisition of relevant competencies through social relationships and interactions that students develop within education, as well as through first-hand knowledge of professional and managerial occupations. Because of the first-hand knowledge and experience offered by placements, some students may think they have an advantage over other students if they should apply to the same organisation for work. But this is not always the case, because employers are particularly concerned that students do not take a passive attitude to demonstrating their competencies and how these relate to the vision of the organisation. Indeed, they may tend to expect more from a potential applicant who has undertaken a placement with them.

What can be done?

Some health and social care schools have given students a day of incorporating their formal learning with a brief look at the workplace. This often combines a programme on the application procedure and curriculum vitae (CV) writing with an interview skills programme, often played by two professionals. In this instance, it is generally believed that any workplace learning programme is enough to help students with a successful transition into employment. However, it does not necessarily provide students with the direct experience required to become experts in the recruitment process. This is because students are not given the hands-on experience needed to gain such expertise. In addition, students have not been given the reflection period required to interweave this area of learning into any practical application before the end of their course.

Time out given for employment-focused reflective practice is vital for gaining an understanding of what is being learnt, as well as how the specific elements of experiences and their ensuing outcomes can be clearly identified, so that experience may be evaluated. This helps identify what we have learnt in order to construct new or different approaches to our future practice, or to recognise and validate effective practice to utilise in the future (Eraut, 1994). Thus, in identifying that learning comes from different incidents and experiences in life, students' thoughts need to be focused on learning much more about themselves, others, their job, the organisation they are applying to work for and their professional practice, as well as their abilities and skills (Eraut, 1994).

In this manner, reflective practice enables students to examine and explore all relevant issues of concern, which are triggered by their individual experiences, and allows clarity in meaning and terms of self that allows changes to take place (Boyd & Fales, 1983). Given that a side-effect of self-reflection is often disquiet and possible uncomfortable feelings, it is important that students challenge these perceptions, place them within a given context and initiate appropriate action through analysis and interpretation to deal with forthcoming issues.

It cannot be emphasised enough that students also need to realise the importance of demonstrating that the knowledge they are applying is not just descriptive but focused upon the critical analysis of practical situations. Boyd and Fales (1983) suggest it is this which gives individuals the depth of understanding and critical analysis needed to deal with different situations. It is also this process of analysis and synthesis that employers look for from their employees. Everything considered, in particular where the employer is concerned, the recruitment process is driven by the desire to find the right person for the job. It is designed to identify people who not only have the right mix of skills and experience but who also aspire to the employer's values. It is very important that the employer therefore gets the recruitment process right, which means that the health and social care employment sector is no more an employee's market but is employer-led.

If students are not already been aware of this, the prospect of facing a competitive employment market means that they will naturally experience a daunting time while negotiating their transition into employment. It is for this reason that developing appropriate strategies at university is useful from an early stage (Clouder & Dalley, 2002).

Raising students' awareness of the recruitment process

In any presentation or lecture that raises awareness of the recruitment process in health and social care, there is always an emphasis on knowledge, learning and experience drawn from the academic context. This is characterised by evidence-based research and its application to practice, through collaboration between professionals to improve care for patients or clients. Additionally, there is usually discussion of the personal context in which students not only have to demonstrate their generic competence to do the job, but where they also have to learn to market their self-conviction and their guiding principles. Information has to be elicited from a whole range of experiences and perceptions and applied to the job as well as to the organisation they will be working for.

As competition is fiercely increasing in the health and social care employment sector, it puts more pressure on the new professional graduates to demonstrate that they are the best person for any post that may become vacant in the NHS. At their best, graduates will also need to draw out of their hat other personal qualities that may help them to get the job. This could include extracurricular interests, achievements and talents that are considered as employability investments which have matured and are ready to be cashed in to kick start their future career. It is this extra 'something' that often allows a graduate to stand above the rest if they are comparably as good as everyone else.

Another approach is to deliver professional practice modules alongside the more theoretical ones, so that students will obtain an enrichment of skills and knowledge, which will not only enable them to become proficient practitioners but will also enhance their learning and personal development through analysis and synthesis. Faust and Faust (2006) refer to this technique as 'Pitch Yourself', as it is this which impinges upon the unique elements of a person.

Raising awareness of the competency-based employer approach

Employers often take a competency-based approach to employment which requires candidates to evidence their get-up-and-go skills, their leadership abilities, their social confidence, problem solving and communication skills. Faust and Faust (2006) claim that, in the initial stages of their application, candidates should demonstrate their potential future performance in the workplace. Rather than thinking 'What can the employer offer me?, it is important to change hats for a moment and ask the question 'What can I offer the employer?'

Obviously, this question can only be answered effectively by researching the employer beforehand to identify what specific skills and attributes are required which can then be demonstrated by the candidate. This match can only be spotted if the individual concerned knows themselves well and is confident in what he or she has to offer.

Making the application count

The mechanism that now governs formal employment application is on-line technology. This again is an example of a recruitment change that has hit the health and social care sector, and it means that information has to be formatted into a specific shape. If the written application does not fit the given format or the technology cannot translate it then the application is rejected. This has almost replaced the traditional hand-written paper application. However, from the employer's viewpoint, it provides a much easier way of short-listing candidates in a competitive and congested job market. It has been suggested that one way of embedding these essential employment application skills at an early stage of health and social care education is to allow students to simulate the work environment through applying for clinical placements while at university; where they will be learning the necessary skills within the safety of their education environment (Harvey & Green, 1994).

By moving the system away from ready-made options to one where health and social care employers and the universities can work together to ensure that students begin to realise the competitive nature of the market, they will also be given the opportunity from an early stage to learn to compete within it. In so doing, students will be prevented from becoming intimidated and nervous about applying for jobs and attending interviews.

Summary of necessary measures

It has been argued that universities need to begin to introduce a number of measures to help tackle the problem that health and social care students have in preparing themselves for the world of work and in applying successfully for scarce jobs.

Firstly, it is necessary to place greater emphasis on helping students to integrate in their minds the experiences and skills they have developed not just on their courses but from their placements. Students need help from lecturers and others to bundle these experiences together so that they can use them coherently as a weapon in their quest for a job.

Aside from this, universities must start to help students learn how to construct better applications for jobs and to deal more effectively with interview situations. This may mean running through 'dummy' applications and interviews individually with students in an environment that is as close to reality as possible. Importantly, students must not just be allowed to go through these simulations and forget them – they need to be offered feedback on how they have performed and how they can improve. They must also be encouraged to reflect on how they have done, with the opportunity to go through the application and/or interview process again if necessary.

One way of reinforcing these simulations would be for higher education institutions to require students to arrange their own placements where possible, rather than do the work for them, thus helping them to cultivate and develop essential skills which will be required when actually applying for a job. However, if in the future students are to apply for clinical placements themselves, then adequate support is needed, not just from academic staff but also from employers, who must be both receptive and supportive of this new kind of placement application procedure, treating it as if it were a graduate appointment. In this way, the process will be rigorous enough for students to learn valuable lessons.

Furthermore, academic staff should also encourage students to make more use of their institution's careers service, which can help them significantly with advice on CV writing, job applications and interview techniques.

At a strategic level, there needs to be a sensible power balance between academic institutions and employers, in which both parties are able to make their views and needs known, so that they can work together in a genuine partnership that satisfies both sides. My impression is that the balance has switched slightly too far towards the needs of employers, so that universities are sometimes afraid to make the NHS aware of what their students needs are. If universities are more assertive, then there will be a benefit to employers, because the likelihood is that they will produce potential employees who are more useful to the NHS. Bringing in all these measures does not require a huge amount of extra resources, merely a change in thinking.

Conclusion

Health and social care graduates are now waking up to the changes that have occurred around them. They can no longer be complacent that they will enter their professional niche based only on the knowledge and skills that have prepared them for entering their relevant professional area. They now need to focus more not only on their reflective practice but on the individual interpersonal skills they will be transferring into the professional arena. Additionally, they need to take into consideration the employer's requirements. They need to give the employer exactly what the employing organisation is looking for. As such, newly qualified professionals in health and social care should constantly ask themselves the questions 'What is this employer looking for?', 'Am I offering the employer what is required?' Graduates will need to explore the depths of their skills, knowledge and experiences and create an impact through relevant evidence, in order to win the competitive battle for getting into that valued profession.

In part this requires a change in mindset from students, but to help engender this, higher education institutions must intervene more decisively to prepare students for the world of work. This means helping them integrate their experiences and skills more meaningfully, allowing them to practise job applications and interviews with appropriate feedback, and encouraging students to arrange placements themselves so that they get some idea of what it takes to secure a job. It also means that institutions must develop genuine partnerships with employers so that the needs of students can be aligned with the needs of the UK's NHS and the primary care trusts.

The application process

The job market

Few jobs are now conventionally advertised within professional journals or the press, but more frequently appear on-line; often with strict guidelines for accepted completion and submission of the application. Graduates must remain vigilant and regularly check for newly posted vacancies; these may be found on the websites of each healthcare professional's representative organisation, plus websites for individual hospital trusts and community-based organisations and schemes. Some hospitals still organise and run open days for new graduates. Often attendance at an open day may be a prerequisite for subsequent application to that healthcare trust. Perhaps more importantly, students must learn to market themselves adequately, starting throughout their clinical training. A successful clinical placement, establishing a good rapport with clinical supervisors, may provide early warning of a vacant post, plus the potential for a valuable clinical reference.

Places to look for jobs include:

▨ various NHS jobs in UK www.nhscareers.nhs.uk;
▨ NHS Professionals www.nhsprofessionals.nhs.uk;
▨ Health Professionals www.healthprofessionals.com;
▨ www.csp.org.uk;
▨ www.cot.org.uk;
▨ www.gscc.org.uk;
▨ local NHS trusts.

It is advisable if possible to gain experience and further training before moving into the private sector.

The application process

Once a potential job has been advertised, it is essential to read the job description very carefully before starting the application process. The personal specification states basic requirements of the job and guides the short listing process.

> Always look at the job description and match your application to the skills required

The strength of the application will determine whether the candidate is shortlisted. Most healthcare institutions will look within the application to identify a list of specific criteria which meet their requirements. Key points to stress include:

▨ why you are interested in working for this particular employer;
▨ what appeals to you about the job;
▨ what you can offer as a candidate;
▨ your commitment and enthusiasm;
▨ professional awareness.

Curriculum vitae

A CV gives a concise summary of an applicant's professional background and experience. It allows the applicant to highlight key experiences, achievements and qualities in order to promote themselves as the most appropriate candidate for the post. A CV is the first thing a potential employer reads about an applicant, from which a large number of assumptions can be made. It is not only the content of a CV which is evaluated; the organization, clarity and formatting of the document also provide valuable information to the potential employer about the applicant. Therefore, the writing of a CV needs careful thought and consideration so that an appropriate impression is made.

Key points to consider:

- Keep CV content to two sides of A4 paper maximum.
- Print CV on good quality paper.
- Use simple layout with clear formatting.
- Avoid excess use of fonts, bold type, underlining and punctuation.
- Make it easy to read.
- Check thoroughly for typographical errors and mistakes.

Always remember that a CV is written with reference to a specific job application; as such it should be adapted for each new job to highlight and stress the appropriate experiences and qualities which match those described in the job description and person specification.

Key points to include in CV are:

- personal details;
- education and qualifications;
- awards;
- professional body membership;
- research;
- publications;
- clinical placement experience;
- previous employment;
- other activities;
- referees.

For the new healthcare graduate, emphasis should be placed on describing their clinical placement experiences; at this level delivery of this information is often used to distinguish between applicants. When recounting previous employment, briefly describe the main duties, but emphasise the transferable skills gained undertaking this work which may be useful in the current application, such as communication skills, team-working experience, and the ability to delegate and carry out accurate documentation.

The 'other activities' section gives the applicant an opportunity to reveal a little more about themselves and highlight other skills and achievements. These may include sporting accolades, travel, and an ability to speak a second language or voluntary work.

It is usual to identify two key people who are willing to provide a written reference. Applicants often select a tutor or faculty member from their training institution who can provide an academic reference. It is helpful if the other referee has a clinical background and can report from a practical viewpoint. Always approach the referee before identifying them on a CV to ask whether they are prepared to write a reference on your behalf and later follow-up by informing them of the application outcome.

This is a fictional CV which provides just one example from the many CV styles in use. Use it as a template to apply your experiences to a specific job.

Alice Walker
60 Hanover Road
Uxbridge, Middlesex
UB8 3PH

E-mail alice@orange.com
Home number 000 0000 0000
Mobile number 00000 000000

Education

2002–2005 BSc (Hons) Physiotherapy (2:1) Brunel University, Middlesex
2001–2002 A level Biology (Grade A) Goodyear College
1987–1990 BA (Hons) Economics (2:1) Essex University

Professional Membership

HPC number 00000
CSP number 00000

Clinical Experience

Care of the Elderly Mental Health Ealing Hospital 6 weeks
Student Physiotherapy key learning points

- Schizophrenia case presentation
- Autonomous management of elderly mental health patient caseload in an inpatient setting and holistic multidisciplinary ('MDT') Community Mental Health Team
- Lead community exercise group and individual hydrotherapy sessions

Outpatients St Bartholomew's Hospital 6 weeks
Student Physiotherapy key learning points

▨ Weekly open assessment clinics
▨ Joint goal setting
▨ Managing exercise classes; back school and knee classes
▨ Time and diary management

Neurology Chelsea & Westminster Hospital 4 weeks
Student Physiotherapy key learning points

▨ Patient and carers education regarding pathology and prognosis
▨ Autonomous ward management and prioritisation
▨ Respond to constructive feedback

Respiratory ITU/HDU and medical ward St. Thomas' Hospital 4 weeks
Student Physiotherapy key learning points

▨ ITU/HDU assessment and treatment techniques e.g. suction: closed and open, positioning and exercise, and management of patients post cardio-thoracic surgery and with Multiple organ failure
▨ Autonomous surgical and medical ward management including risk assessment
▨ Cardiac rehabilitation delivery involvement
▨ Use of intermittent positive pressure breathing equipment
▨ Appreciation gained of weaning from mechanical ventilation, ITU drugs and non-invasive ventilation

Regional Neurosurgery Unit Charing Cross Hospital 4 weeks
Student Physiotherapy key learning points

▨ Brain tumour case presentation and lead weekly journal club
▨ Acute brain injury patient management post neurosurgery including hoist and tilt table use
▨ Applying and monitoring splints inspiring 3rd year research project regarding splint efficacy

Out Patients Bolingbroke Hospital 4 weeks
Student Physiotherapy key learning points

▨ Sub-acromial impingement syndrome case presentation
▨ Patient assessment techniques
▨ Designing and progressing individual treatment plans including home exercise programmes
▨ Electrotherapy, joint mobilisation and palpation skills

Orthopedics trauma and elective wards St Mary's Hospital 4 weeks
Student Physiotherapy key learning points

▪ Lead physiotherapy team anatomy seminars plus fractured neck of femur case presentation
▪ Autonomous ward management
▪ MDT home visits to assess patient function and exercise in home environment

Respiratory ITU/surgical ward West Middlesex University Hospital 4 weeks
Student Physiotherapy key learning points

▪ ITU assessment and treatment techniques including rehabilitation of maxil-lofacial surgery and long-term ITU patients
▪ Autonomous surgical ward management
▪ Pulmonary rehabilitation delivery
▪ Arterial blood gas analysis and X-ray analysis skills
▪ Appreciation gained of CPAP and Trache care

Skills Profile
Communication

▪ Verbal and non-verbal communication skills enhanced by communication with a chronic stroke patient with limited vocabulary due to expressive dysphasia. Engagement of a speech and language therapist determined the patient could comprehend speech and use 'yes', 'no' and non-verbal gestures to communicate effectively. The patient agreed goals and engaged in rehabilitation in partnership with myself.
▪ Clear and concise medical and physiotherapy notes affording effective and efficient communication with the MDT.
▪ Patient case studies and in-service training delivered to physiotherapy and occupational therapy teams including seniors, juniors and assistants. Presentation via PowerPoint slides supported by handouts.

Teamwork

▪ Orthopaedic placement experience allowed engagement in MDT joint goal setting, including mobilisation reinforced by nursing staff and occupational therapists, and discharge planning with joint home assessment visits conducted.
▪ Teach and manage physiotherapy assistants to assist in the delivery of neurology treatment plans. Skills taught to assistants included supporting stroke patients in standing to facilitate reaching forward and picking objects up.

Problem solving and clinical reasoning

▪ On respiratory placement I encountered a patient on a surgical ward who was pyrexic, had SaO_2 below normal parameters and had retained secretions indicating respiratory compromise post-op. Using clinical reasoning

I re-positioned the patient from slump lying to high sitting, taught the Active Cycle of Breathing, sent a sputum sample for analysis and requested that the registrar consider antibiotics for a chest infection.

Computer

▪ Knowledge of Microsoft Office and use of Word, PowerPoint and Excel for in-service presentations.

Previous Employment
1996–2002 Senior Manager, Accountant, Deliotte, London.
1991–1996 Accountant, Grant Thornton, London.
Feb–Sept 2002 Volunteer Physiotherapy Assistant, Outpatients, Bolingbroke Hospital. One day per week including hydrotherapy and clinical notes audit.

Hobbies
Playing badminton and five-a-side football, travelling, socialising with friends, cinema and reading.

References
Provided on request

The interview

The purpose of the interview from the perspective of an organisation is to find out if the candidate lives up to the claims made on the application. Specifically, whether the candidate meets the core requirements of the job and can offer supporting evidence of this. The interview also provides a forum to assess the candidate's interpersonal skills and whether they will fit well into the team, department and the organisation.

For the interviewee, it is an opportunity to market and 'sell yourself' for the job; but at the same time find out more about the post and the culture of the organisation. It is very important to be able to answer the question 'Do I really want to work for this organisation?'

Given the growing number of applications received for any given junior healthcare professional post, organisations are frequently holding assessment exercises as part of a selection process, in order to identify which candidates will proceed to attend a face-to-face interview.

Assessment exercises

These might include:

▪ written clinical scenario;
▪ watch a video and assess a patient video;
▪ carry out a task in a team;
▪ told beforehand about a presentation.

Face-to face interview

The interview is usually conducted by at least two or three personnel, one of whom may be a representative from human resources. Each in turn will ask the candidate questions from several categories:

- Opening or personal questions:
  - Justify career choice
  - What is your greatest achievement?
  - What skills can you bring to this job?
- Clinical or practical questions:
  - How to treat patient with particular condition
  - Justify prioritorisation for treatment of three different patients
  - Explain considerations when discharging patient into the community
- Questions relating to professionalism:
  - What is meant by term CPD?
  - What is the role of the regulating professional body?
  - How may knowledge and skills framework influence your intervention?
- Problem-solving scenarios:
  - Give an example of appropriate delegation of work
  - You are in a situation where a team isn't working. What can you do?
  - What skills and qualities can you bring to a team?
- Communication issues:
  - What makes a good communicator?
  - What would you do if a colleague was having problems that could affect their work and patients?
- Topical or political change:
  - How does your healthcare profession contribute to the health and well being of the general public?
  - Give an example of how evidence-based practice has influenced your work
  - How do the financial strains on this institution affect your profession?

Use the job description and person specification to identify 'obvious' questions and prepare thorough answers. It is an extremely useful exercise to practise answering questions out loud, as it is often difficult to formulate a coherent response from ideas when under pressure during the interview. The key to a successful outcome is adequate preparation; it is very apparent to an interview panel which candidates have taken the time to think about the job opportunity and prepare appropriately.

It is expected that an interviewee may be nervous during the interview process. Therefore, take time to collect thoughts and structure an appropriate response rather than trying to answer the question immediately. It is perfectly acceptable to ask for a question to be repeated if necessary. When the interview panel has completed their questions, there is usually an opportunity for the candidate to ask questions about the job or the organisation. Try to identify at least three pertinent questions to ask the panel; if the answer to a question has been covered elsewhere then inform them of that and move on to the next question on the list.

Attending an interview is a valuable learning experience independent of outcome. Therefore, on leaving the interview reflect on your performance in order to identify areas of strength and weakness, highlighting areas which can be developed and improved. After completion of the interview aim to write down all the questions asked by the panel, so they can be used again in preparation for a subsequent interview.

Key self-assessment points include:

▨ Did you do yourself justice?
▨ Could you have improved your performance? How?
▨ Were you properly prepared?
▨ Which questions did you answer well?
▨ Which questions did you struggle with?
▨ Were any gaps in your skills or experience revealed?

Employer's criticism of interview performance

The interview panel will adhere to strict criteria when evaluating a candidate's performance. Often a scoring system is used to identify the key points required for an acceptable answer. However, despite having a broad knowledge base, candidates are also simultaneously assessed on their interpersonal skills, attitude and presentation; often it is these elements that contribute to an unsuccessful outcome. If an interview has been unsuccessful, always ask the institution for feedback as to why, so these issues may be addressed for the next opportunity. Common criticism from employers of interview performance includes the following areas:

▨ candidate didn't do good enough self-marketing;
▨ candidate didn't elaborate on responses to questions;
▨ candidate was dull and/or lacked enthusiasm;
▨ poor interpersonal skills/looked away all the time;
▨ couldn't discuss or support items listed on CV;
▨ candidate didn't know anything about specific hospital/healthcare institution;
▨ candidate spoke too much, not allowing interviewers to speak;
▨ candidate appeared unprofessional or unprepared.

Interview tips

Attending an interview for the first time can be a daunting experience. However, it is important to remember the interview process has a dual purpose; it gives the candidate an opportunity to gain further information about the job on offer and the employing institution, and offers the institution an opportunity to assess the candidate's suitability for the post. Therefore, the interviewers aim to facilitate the best from the candidate, and are not trying to expose areas of weakness.

Key points for a successful outcome include:

- Treat every interview as though it is a formal business presentation and the product you are selling is yourself.
- Get the correct balance in terms of confidence and arrogance.
- Read the professional press so you are aware of latest professional issues relevant to healthcare.
- Be proactive in mentioning topical issues in the interview; don't wait to be asked.
- Make eye contact with the interviewer when answering a question.
- Smile and be friendly.
- Reflect good body language.

References

Ayas, K., Zenuick, N. (2001) Project based learning: building communities of reflective practitioners. *Management Learning* **32**(1), 61–76.

Barbieri, P. (2003) Social capital and self employment: a network analysis experiment and several considerations. *International Sociology* **8**(4), 681–701.

Barker, K., Bosco, C., Oandansa, I.F. (2005) Factors in implementing interprofessional education and collaborative practice initiatives: findings from key informant interviews. *Journal of Interprofessional Practice* **S1**, 166–176.

Barnitt, R., Salmond, R. (2000) Fitness for purpose of occupational therapy graduates: two different perspectives. *British Journal of Occupational Therapy* **63**(9), 443–448.

Barr, H. (2000) New NHS, new collaboration, new agenda for education. *Journal of Professional Care* **14**(1), 81–86.

Barr, H., Hammick, M., Koppel, I., Reeves, S. (1999) Evaluating interprofessional education: two systematic reviews for health and social care. *British Education Research Journal* **25**(4), 533–544.

Bate, P., Robert, G., Bevan, H. (2004) The next phase of healthcare improvement: what can we learn from social movements? *Quality and Safety in Health Care* **13**(1), 62–64.

Boyd, E.M., Fales A.W. (1983) Reflective learning: key to learning from experience. *Journal of Humanistic Psychology* **23**(2), 99–117.

Brunel University (2003/04) *The destinations of graduate statistics.* UK: Brunel University.

Callaghan, J. (1976) *Towards a National Debate.* Speech by Prime Minister James Callaghan at a foundation stone laying ceremony at Ruskin College Oxford, England.

Clouder, L., Dalley, J. (2002) Providing a 'safety net': fine tuning preparation of undergraduate physiotherapists for contemporary professional practice. *Learning in Health and Social Care* **1**(4), 191–201.

Cooper, H., Spencer-Dawe, E. (2006) Involving service users in interprofessional education narrowing the gap between theory and practice. *Journal of Interprofessional Care* **20**(6), 603–617.

Cooper, H., Spencer-Dawe, E., McLean, E. (2005) Beginning the process of teamwork: design, implementation and evaluation of an inter-professional education intervention for first year undergraduate students. *Journal of Interprofessional Care* **19**(5), 492–508.

D'eon M (2005) A blueprint for Interprofessional learning. *Journal of Interprofessional Care* **S1**, 49–59.

Davys, D., Pope, K. (2006) Problem-based learning within occupational therapy education: a summary of the Salford experience. *British Journal of Occupational Therapy* **69**(12), 572–574.

Dearing, R. (1997) *The Dearing Report: National Committee of Inquiry into Higher Education. Higher Education in the Learning Society*. London: HMSO.

Duffy, F.D., Gordon, G.H., Whelan, G., Cole-Kelly, K., Frankel, R. (2004) Assessing competence in communication and interpersonal skills: the Kalamazoo 11 Report. *Academic Medicine* **79**(6), 495–507.

Eraut, M. (1994) *Developing Professional Knowledge and Competence*. UK: Falmer Press.

Faust, B., Faust, M. (2006) *Pitch Yourself*, 2nd edn. London: Pearson Prince Hall Business.

Freeth, D., Hammick, M., Reeves, S., Koppel, I., Barr, H. (2005) *Effective Interpersonal Education. Development Delivery and Evaluation*. Oxford: Blackwell Publishing.

Gelmont, S.B., White, A.W., Carlson, L., Norman, L. (2000) Making organizational change to achieve improvement and interprofessional learning: perspectives from health professional educators. *Journal of Interprofessional Care* **14**(2), 131–146.

Hammick, M. (2000) Interprofessional education: evidence from the past to guide the future. *Medical Teacher* **22**(5), 466–467

Harvey, L., Green, D. (1994) *Employer Satisfaction*. Birmingham: QHE.

Harvey, L., Moon, S., Geall, V. (1997) Graduates' work: organisational change and students' attributes. Birmingham: The University of Central England, Centre for Research into Quality.

Her Majesty's Stationery Office (1963) *Higher Education: the report of the committee under the chairmanship of Lord Robbins*. Cm 2154. London: HMSO.

Hilton, R., Morris, J. (2001) Student placements – is there evidence supporting team skill development in clinical practice?*Journal of Interprofessional Care* **15**(2), 171–183.

Holmes, L. (2000) Reframing the skills agenda in higher education and the double warrant. Paper, presented at a conference on The Future Business of Higher Education. Lady Margaret Hall, Oxford.

Iliffe, S., Munroe, J. (2000) New Labour and Britain's National Health Service: an overview of current reforms. *International Journal of Health Services* **30**(2), 309–334.

Jarvis, P. (2006) Teaching styles and teaching method. In: P Jarvis (ed) *The Theory and Practice of Teaching*. London: Routledge Taylor & Francis Group.

Leitch, S. (2005) *Skills in the UK: The Long-Term Challenge*. London: HMSO.

Lewis, R., Gillam, S. (2001) The National Health Service Plan: further reform of British health care? *International Journal of Health and Social Services* **13**(1), 111–118.

Mann, S. (2005) A health-care model of emotional labour: an evaluation of the literature and development of a model. *Journal of Health Organization and Management* **19**(5), 304–317.

McCluskey, A., Cusick, A. (2002) Strategies for introducing evidence-based practice and changing clinician behaviour. A manager's toolbox. *Australian Occupational Therapy* **49**(2), 63–70.

Nybø, G. (2004) Personnel development for dissolving jobs: towards a competency-based approach? *International Journal of Human Resource Management* **15**(3), 549–564.

Perkins, D., Salomon, G. (1994) Transfer of learning. In: T. Husen, T. Postlethwaite (eds) *The International Encyclopaedia of Education*. Oxford: Pergamon.

Regan De Bere, S. (2003) Evaluating the implications of complex interprofessional education for improvements in collaborative practice: a multidimensional model. *British Educational Research Journal* **29**(1), 105–124.

Sparrow, P.R. (2007) Globalization of HR at function level: four UK-based case studies of the international recruitment and selection process. *International Journal of Human Resource Management* **18**(5), 845–867.

Sutton, G., Griffin, M.A. (2000) Transition from students to practitioner: the role of expectations, values and personality. *British Journal of Occupational Therapy* **63**(8), 380–388.

University Grants Committee (1984) *A Strategy for Higher Education into the 1990s: The University Grants Committee's Advice*. London: Her Majesty's Stationery Office.

Webb, S. (2001) Some considerations on the validity of evidence-based practice in social workers. *British Journal of Social Work* **31**(1), 57–79.

White Paper (1987) *Higher Education: Meeting the Challenge*. London: Her Majesty's Stationery Office.

Wilcock, P.M., Headrick, L.A. (2000) Interprofessional learning for the improvement of health care: why bother? *Journal of Interprofessional Care* **14**(2), 111–117.

12: Career planning for therapists

Christine Craik

Introduction

A few years ago, there would have been little interest in a chapter on career planning for therapists in the UK. There was a plentiful choice of posts for graduates and later, when seeking a senior post, there were enticing advertisements extolling the benefits of working for a wide variety of employers. Many therapists chose to work in the NHS, with some moving to other areas of employment due to a steady expansion in career opportunities. More recently there has been a change in the job market for therapists in the UK with a reduction in the number of junior posts, particularly in physiotherapy.

The realities of the workplace, evident for other professions, are now affecting therapists. But therapists in other countries also face uncertainty. Where the professions are well established there have also been fluctuations in the job market, while in countries where the professions are still developing, the challenge can be to persuade employers of the benefits of the therapy professions. Although this appears daunting, it may provide a stimulus for the professions and individual therapists to expand their practice into new areas beyond the comforts and confines of a traditional NHS career. However, occupational therapy and physiotherapy would not have developed to their current position without the vision and determination of their founders and subsequent skill and enterprise of the leaders who have guided the professions. The challenges of current times, which initially seem to be portents of misfortune, may be the impetus to take the professions to the next stage of their development.

This chapter explores the traditional therapy career path, examines the changes influencing it and contemplates future possibilities. It considers embarking on a therapy career and alternatives to rotational posts, and then it examines progressing from a first post and career development. In a rapidly developing environment, current information is important and so throughout this chapter consulting key websites and current publications is recommended for timely advice.

Setting the scene

Traditional career path

Previously, career planning for most therapists in the UK was straight-forward. On successful completion of a degree programme, there were many junior posts, usually in the NHS. Most therapists had a choice of locations to work and many opted to start their career in a rotational post providing several months' experience in a variety of practice areas. This was an opportunity to consolidate learning, to experience working in a range of settings with different clients groups and to assist in selecting an area for future specialisation. After a few years, therapists would apply for a senior post in their chosen area and, with a shortage of staff, there was often little competition. Further promotion was often easily obtained as the shortages were more critical at senior levels. There were openings beyond health and social care with therapists opting for private practice, research, education or management, in addition to those who pursued highly specialised clinical posts.

Recent changes

Around 2004 the situation changed initially for physiotherapists and, later, and to a lesser extent, for occupational therapists, due to an imbalance between supply and demand. Since the inception of the professions, demand for therapists has exceeded supply. As the education of therapists in England and Wales is funded by the NHS, they have controlled supply. As a result of patient influence, lobbying by the professions and Department of Health Policy, the NHS financed a steady increase in student numbers until the late 1990s. Then in response to the NHS Plan (Department of Health, 2000a), the numbers increased significantly, creating additional graduates from 2003. Then there were indications that increases had been too great with the Health Care Workforce (2005) recommending that the number of occupational therapy students should remain constant at least until the 2006 intake but there should be a small reduction in physiotherapy students due to the possible over supply and the reported difficulty of physiotherapy graduates in obtaining posts (Craik, 2006). Subsequently in 2006 and 2007, the NHS reduced funding for students and there may be further reductions. Professional organisations and others have warned of the long-term hazards of this policy as once the number of students is reduced, it will take many years to reverse the trend.

The situation has been compounded by financial cutbacks in the NHS to balance budgets, reducing the number of junior posts especially for physiotherapists. It is not clear if this apparent decrease in demand for therapists is a real measure of patient need or is a manifestation of reduced funding. Conversely, there are indications that requirements for therapy services will grow with the increasing survival rates of premature babies, and policies enabling people with disabilities back to employment and facilitating older people to remain at home. These changes, coupled with an ageing workforce due to retire over the next decade, will increase the demand for therapists. Anticipating these changes and future patterns of service delivery may indicate future job opportunities.

Future patterns of service delivery

There has been a steady move from acute inpatient provision to day and community services provided by the NHS and social services, and this trend will continue with the creation of polyclinics first proposed for London (NHS London, 2007). Increasingly there will be a move to provision by the private sector, including private practice, and also by the third sector, which operates between the public and private sector and includes charities, foundations and voluntary organisations (Department of Health, 2006). It has been suggested that occupational therapists will move more into health promotion (College of Occupational Therapists, 2002) and, in a paper exploring ways to increase posts for healthcare graduates, the Department of Health (2007) suggests potential new roles for the professions in occupational health, especially for physiotherapists in musculoskeletal practice.

Impact on therapy careers

There will be fewer posts for therapists in acute services in the NHS, although this may be offset by a move to more generic working creating other opportunities. When there was a shortage of therapists, they tended to retain their professional role. Indeed, there has been apparent disapproval of therapists who pursued this route as though they were abandoning their profession. The therapists who made this transition have often been successful, as the knowledge and attributes which make proficient therapists are transferable to other roles. However, they have a responsibility to maintain their professional focus and to promote their professional origin to others and raise the profile of the professions. Perhaps some therapists have not done this in the past, being apprehensive of the disapproval of therapy colleagues. However, if the move to a more generic post is part of a career pathway and not permanent, then retaining a professional focus, membership of the professional body and registration with the Health Professions Council will be essential to enable transition back into a therapy post.

Within social services, the number of posts may be maintained or expanded. Although the move to service users controlling their own budgets will change the role of staff in the social care sector. Occupational therapists have been employed in this sector since the legislative changes in the 1960s and 1970s. Although the number of occupational therapists employed is smaller than social workers, they play a significant role with many clients, especially those with complex disabilities. Here, promotion for occupational therapists is again likely to involve a move to a more generic post of team leader.

As services transfer to the third sector, there will be a need for the therapy professions to increase their visibility there. Although only a small proportion of therapists have worked in this sector, some have made an exceptional impact. Elizabeth Fanshawe, an occupational therapist and wheelchair user due to childhood polio, was employed by the Disabled Living Foundation from 1970. She became its Director in 1983 and was awarded an OBE in 1985 for her services to disabled people (College of Occupational Therapists, 2004). In the past, voluntary organisations and charities may have wanted to employ therapists but the higher salaries offered in the NHS may have prevented this. Now in a more competitive market, therapists may be more willing to consider these options.

Private sector provision has increased, especially in some specialities. This has created additional occupational therapy posts in forensic mental health and more physiotherapy posts in elective orthopaedics and this trend is set to continue. Physiotherapists have a more established position in private practice than occupational therapists, but here too there have been developments in recent years and this is likely to continue.

Future career paths

It seems likely that the familiar therapy career path of a rotation post followed by a more senior post and then specialisation in the NHS will become less common. This has implications, not only for students and graduates, but also for the academics and supervisors who advise them and the managers who will employ them. Lateral thinking, flexibility and creativity will be required by everyone involved and the professional organisations have an important lobbying and leadership role.

A future career pathway might be a physiotherapy graduate who wants to specialise in paediatrics. On graduation, she cannot obtain a physiotherapy post, so following CSP guidance she becomes a volunteer overseas with a charity for children with neurological problems. Six months later, on return to the UK, her experience leads to a physiotherapy post with the same charity. After a year, recognising that she is working in the third sector in a specialised area, she begins part-time study on a Master's programme in physiotherapy. The following year she is successful in obtaining an NHS band 5 post and on completion of her preceptorship year, she is promoted to band 6. Her studies continue and, when considering her dissertation, she discusses with her manager a topic that would be valuable to the service, meet the academic requirement of her degree and enhance her knowledge of paediatrics. On graduation from her degree, she is successful in a lateral move to a band 6 post in the children's service of the same trust. The following year, she is promoted to band 7 in the same service and she can see her future career in this service progressing to clinical specialist or perhaps a consultant therapist post.

An alternative career pathway could be an occupational therapy graduate from a 4-year part-time programme who continues working part-time for the NHS mental health trust that sponsored her. On graduation, she completes her preceptorship year in a forensic setting. But, after seven years working for the trust she wants a change and she obtains a post in a private hospital for forensic mental health patients. Here she enjoys the challenge and benefits of the private sector but, after 2 years, she wants to extend her knowledge and moves back to the NHS to a band 6 post in a community mental health team. Here, her generic skills are extended, but after a year she wants to develop her occupational therapy knowledge and so she enrolls on a part time MSc occupational therapy course. At the end of her first year, she obtains a band 7 post in a rehabilitation ward for people with enduring mental health problems with the interview panel being impressed by the work she had undertaken for one of her assessments. After 2 years and the completion of her MSc, the post of manager of the rehabilitation ward is advertised and she realises that she meets the person specification; she applies for the post and is successful. She will maintain her Health Professions Council registration and College of Occupational Therapists membership as she sees her long-term future in the profession, but in the meantime she is enjoying the challenge of her new post.

Starting out on a therapy career

Sources of information

Obtaining a first post is challenging for graduates of all disciplines and most universities will have a careers service offering general advice on preparing CVs, and interview preparation and performance. They will do this through their website and many will offer training sessions or individual tutorials.

More specific advice will often be included advice in the physiotherapy and occupational therapy curriculum as individual lectures or as part of a module. Personal or academic tutors or other staff should be consulted for more personal guidance based on their knowledge of individual student performance. While on placement, students should be alert to job opportunities, and placement supervisors may be a source of valuable guidance and can often provide a job reference. Many therapists go on to obtain a first post in a setting or area of practice where they had a placement.

The Chartered Society of Physiotherapy (www.csp.co.uk) and the College of Occupational Therapists (www.cot.co.uk) offer more specific professional advice. While written publications are available, regular visits to their websites will provide up the most up-to-date information in a rapidly changing environment.

Rotational posts

Rotational posts have become an accepted route into the profession for physiotherapists and to a lesser extent for occupational therapists. However, in changing times this will be challenged not only due to the shortage of such posts but also due to the changing profile of graduates. The Chartered Society of Physiotherapy (2003), in its guidance for new entrants to physiotherapy, suggests that obtaining rotation experience is important. While many occupational therapists have opted for a rotational post, some do not and the College of Occupational Therapists has not promoted this as a preferred option. This is probably due to the profession's wider sphere of practice, encompassing mental health and social services. While some rotations have included general and mental health practice, there have been few with NHS and social services combinations, so occupational therapists wishing to specialise in mental health may have commenced their career directly in that setting. Conventionally, few social service departments have recruited graduates, preferring those with some NHS experience, but this has changed recently with more graduates commencing their career there.

The reason for the establishment of rotational posts is interesting. They are now presented as opportunities to assist graduates consolidate their knowledge and skills in a variety of key professional settings in the NHS. By gaining experience in these core areas, graduates are assisted to choose their future career direction. However, there is an alternative perspective. When there was a shortage of graduates, recruitment to less attractive areas of practice was difficult, and managers found that offering a rotation combining these areas with more popular areas was an effective method of recruitment.

To some extent, this reasoning depends on the view that graduates have little previous experience of health and social care, have no identified career goals and require further exposure to more areas of practice to help them decide. This is no longer true, especially in occupational therapy, with many mature students entering the profession with defined career aspirations. They have not viewed a rotation as necessary to their goal. Similarly, there are more part-time students sponsored by their employer for whom they continue to work while studying. On graduation, they usually remain with that employer, bypassing the rotation system.

Alternatives to rotations

While previous advice may have cautioned against early specialisation, the current climate may demand a more pragmatic approach.

If graduates can obtain a post in a specialist area, they would be advised to accept it but to be mindful of potential disadvantages. Those who embark on a specialist route early in their career may wish to use continuing professional development opportunities to maintain a broader focus to enhance their practice and prepare for future opportunities in other areas.

Some graduates with previous experience or with a career plan may seek and find a therapy post in their chosen area of practice in their preferred location. However, first choices may not be available, so there may be a need to think more widely. As some areas of practice may be less attractive, applying for a post there may be more successful. Thinking of less conventional routes to an eventual career ambition may also be productive. If posts are available in a less popular area previously seen as specialist, then working there may be a useful starting point for a more general career. Some practice areas are useful as a crossover to another. So working in a rehabilitation ward for older adults can be a gateway to rehabilitation of other client groups, rehabilitation in the community or specialising in active ageing.

Short- or fixed-term contacts

Sometimes posts are available for a fixed term to cover maternity leave or a secondment or when funding is released for a specific project. They can be a useful starting point and may lead to a more permanent post and, if not, they provide valuable experience. Future employers are likely to view this work experience favourably and making the connection between this and future posts will enhance this experience.

Location

Graduates should consider the location of their first post, as employment patterns vary throughout the UK. While many therapists will be limited to where they are able to work, others may be freer to choose another part of the country with more opportunities. Large cities, especially London, tend to attract graduates, but after a few years many may relocate due to higher house prices and other factors. So there may be less competition for a first post in rural or suburban areas.

Agency working

There are many locum agencies that aim to find employment for those therapists that register with them. Many offer attractive salaries and some offer inducements to register with them. It is advisable to check terms and conditions carefully, as holiday entitlement, benefits and continuing professional development opportunities may be different from traditional employment. However, in a competitive market, they will also find it difficult to obtain posts for graduates.

Part-time work

Although part-time work is most often associated with those with family responsibilities, it could be a short-term option, perhaps combined with another part-time post until a full-time post becomes available. Recent graduates have combined part-time work with part-time postgraduate education, developing work experience and acquiring further educational qualifications that will be of use in future career developments.

Postgraduate education

Although more therapists undertake postgraduate study, most have waited until they have clinical experience. While there are benefits to this route and some courses expect it, if therapy posts are in short supply then starting on a postgraduate qualification on completion of pre-registration education may be a sensible option. A full-time post-registration Master's degree can usually be completed in 1 year and part-time over 2–3 years.

A further option that some therapists may consider is PhD study, usually over 3 years full-time or 4–6 years part-time. A few full-time bursaries may be available from some universities. Although a normal route in other disciplines, it has not previously been attractive to therapists as the limited bursary could not compete with a therapy salary. A note of caution is advised, as two occupational therapists who completed a PhD on graduation reported difficulties when seeking an occupational therapy post (Henderson & Maciver, 2003). However, as postgraduate study at both Master's and Doctoral level has increased, attitudes are likely to change.

A PhD will be necessary for therapists who wish to pursue a research or academic career. So for some therapists who wish to do this, it may be an option to start on this route on graduation, however, some clinical work will be necessary for these routes, so combining this option with some part-time clinical work would be advisable.

First post not in physiotherapy or occupational therapy?

The real challenge is for those who cannot obtain a first post in physiotherapy or occupational therapy. Acquiring a job that uses transferable skills, maintains clinical skills and prepares for a future therapy career has become the goal of some graduates.

Short-term generic or non-therapy posts

An obvious route is short-term employment in a related area while seeking a therapy post. In the UK most students graduate in the summer and seek work from then into the autumn, but later in the year there will be further vacancies as existing staff leave or are promoted. When there are financial constraints, it is often at the end of one financial year around January or at the beginning of next in April that funds are released for additional posts. These may be fruitful times to obtain a therapy post, but gaining relevant employment until then may increase employability.

In choosing a post, it is important to link the knowledge and skills obtained during pre-registration education, the post applied for and the experience to be gained there that will assist in future applications. Thus, therapy assistant posts would be a first choice, but healthcare assistant, rehabilitation assistant and other roles in the NHS would be valuable. Work in social services or the third sector would be other alternatives, and the more imaginative will find other solutions. These posts may be advertised in local newspapers or in the public sector sections of national newspapers. Recent examples have been activities co-ordinator in a day centre for people with mental health problems and support worker for people with learning disabilities living in the community. Some of these posts may operate on a shift system, allowing time for part-time postgraduate study.

Rather than choosing any post, graduates are advised to weigh up alternatives. A physiotherapist wanting to focus on paediatrics but with no relevant placement experience might find it useful to work in a summer camp for disabled children, or someone wanting to specialise in sports physiotherapy could find work in a sport club helpful. An occupational therapist seeking to specialise in learning disabilities might find work in a horticultural charity offering work experience for these clients, while, for another, employment as a welfare rights officer could be useful preparation for an occupational therapy post in social services. Making connections between a short-term post and a future therapy career is important and reflecting on what has been learned and articulating the benefits can transform what may initially seem a negative episode into a more positive one.

Whatever the employment, it is usually easier to move from one post to another and a good reference from a manager who can testify to attitudes to work, team working, attendance and punctuality will be a useful addition to an academic reference. This will be particularly useful for younger graduates with little previous work experience. This approach has been successful for many graduates who have subsequently moved to a therapy post within a matter of months.

If there is no suitable post in related employment then combining a more routine job with postgraduate education or voluntary work in a related area may provide a short-term response. However, volunteering should not be seen as a way of employers obtaining the services of therapists without paying for them as this could be seen as exploiting graduates. So, some voluntary work may be an option, but care must be taken that relevant insurance is in place and that graduates consider what roles they undertake.

Longer-term alternatives

For graduates who do not wish to adopt a short-term strategy until a more permanent post becomes available, other approaches should be considered. Finding an alternative for 1 or 2 years may require a different plan. Again there is a need to connect what has been acquired during pre-registration education to the current post and to future prospects in a therapy career.

Working overseas

Working overseas has previously been recommended only for those with experience in their own country, but it may now be preferable to work in a therapy post whatever its location. Different countries will have different expectations and styles of practice and some may not wish to recruit new graduates. Much will depend on the job market in each country. It has been customary for Australian therapists to come to the UK to work but this has recently been reversed, with a shortage of therapists in some parts of Australia leading to the recruitment of UK therapists there.

Graduates contemplating this option are advised to seek advice from the Chartered Society of Physiotherapy (www.csp.co.uk) or College of Occupational Therapists (www.cot.co.uk). Regulatory and educational requirements vary in different countries and should be checked via the World Confederation for Physical Therapy (http://www.wcpt.org) or the World Federation of Occupational Therapists (http://www.wfot.org.au) and with the intended country. Some countries will require that applicants sit a further examination and there may be issues with the compatibility of qualifications in countries where Master's or Doctoral level qualifications are required.

Volunteering overseas may be another option and the World Federation of Occupational Therapists and the World Confederation for Physical Therapy offer advice on this, as does Voluntary Service Overseas. While they have vacancies for experienced therapists, their Youth for Development programme provides opportunity for young people aged 18–25 to work with VSO for 1 year in a number of countries (http://www.vso.org.uk/volunteering/youth/yfd/index.asp#0). Although this role may not be therapy, working with disadvantaged people in their own countries will provide invaluable experience. The Chartered Society of Physiotherapy offers sensible advice on making the most of these opportunities and recommends maintaining a professional portfolio to provide evidence of learning for the Health Professions Council and future employers (Hobden, 2007).

Non-therapy/generic posts

Longer-term employment in a non-therapy or generic post in a related area can be a gateway to a future therapy career. Here perhaps occupational therapists have an advantage. From the mid 1990s the profession has advocated different models of practice placement and Wood (2005) distinguished between non-traditional placements, where supervision is provided by an occupational therapist, and role-emerging placements in a non-traditional setting, where no occupational therapist is employed. In a survey she reported that 21 of the 24 educational programmes who responded used these new models (Wood, 2005). Totten and Pratt (2001) describe one such placement in a project for homeless people in Glasgow and note that initially these placements were elective but later became standard for all students. As well as making up for a shortfall of placements in conventional settings, it was hoped that this policy would extend the scope of the profession and produce new posts for occupational therapists in these settings. Although to date there has been no research in this area, some universities report that students undertaking such placements may later find employment there. Recent examples include the appointment of the first occupational therapist in a school for disabled children following a successful placement, and the employment of an occupational therapy graduate to a horticultural charity. More recently the Chartered Society of Physiotherapy (2006) has issued guidance on student placements in community and non-traditional settings. Hopefully, this will also lead to new posts.

In seeking such an alternative post, there may be benefits in pursuing work opportunities with a specific client group that will develop knowledge and skills for future therapy posts. There are several generic posts for which a therapy education will provide a useful foundation. Social service and the voluntary sector are likely to provide the most opportunities. Support workers, carers, day centre workers and project worker posts are available with a wide variety of client groups.

Maintaining a professional focus in a generic post

Where therapists start their career in a non-therapy post, retaining a professional focus is essential. Registering with the Health Professions Council is not only advised but may also be obligatory if a generic post has been obtained because of a physiotherapy or occupational therapy qualification. Initial registration on completion of a recognised UK degree programme is more straightforward than attempting to do so later when a period of supervised practice may be required. It will also be important to ensure that the requirements for continuing registration are carried out. This will involve carefully documenting continuing professional development activities and demonstrating their relevance to current or future therapy practice.

Similarly, membership of the College of Occupational Therapists or Chartered Society of Physiotherapy is also highly recommended to keep up to date with the profession and access continuing professional development opportunities and also to provide professional insurance cover. Joining a specialist section of the professional organisation can be another way of maintaining and developing knowledge, as can becoming a committee member or undertaking a volunteering role. The Chartered Society of Physiotherapy has suggested mentorship, further training and understanding about working with scope of practice as further ways to ensure a professional focus in non-NHS posts (Anon, 2007).

Moving on from a first post

Some of the principles identified in obtaining a first post are equally relevant when considering career development. In the future, it is likely that therapists will have more diverse careers, moving in and out of statutory services, perhaps with periods working in the voluntary or private sector. Some may work overseas for a time. Others may combine jobs, in the so-called portfolio career, perhaps working part-time for the NHS and undertaking some private practice or combining clinical work with lecturing or research. Many posts will have more flexibility with therapists perhaps working shifts over a 7-day week. The possibility of therapists working from home for part of the week may become more common. Some therapists may not always work in a post that has occupational therapy or physiotherapy in the title but nevertheless utilises key therapy skills and knowledge. It is likely that the boundaries of professional practice will expand. Preparing for these different opportunities is challenging and demands planning, continuing professional development and maintenance of a professional focus.

NHS employment

For those employed in the NHS, career pathways are more clearly identified with new graduates entering at band 5 and undertaking a preceptorship year with two development reviews and successful completion linked to pay progression (DOH, 2004). Similarly for those remaining within the NHS, there are gateways to progression to higher bands. However, rather than the previous rapid promotion for many therapists, the current scheme anticipates that staff will remain at each band for longer than before. Thus, therapists may have more that one post at each band and may have to consider a lateral move within a band to provide additional experience in another area of practice. Therapists will, therefore, have to manage their career more actively than in the past and think about which post will add to their experience and employability. Here, sound advice is to envisage what employers are seeking rather than what the individual has to offer. Careful scrutiny of job advertisements, job descriptions and person specifications well before applying for a post will provide some guidance. Discussions at performance review with a supervisor or with a mentor will also be valuable.

It is generally accepted that promotion to band 7 will require some evidence of study at Master's level and therapists should think how to incorporate this into their career planning.

The creation of the post of consultant therapist (DOH, 2000a,b) was heralded as a great step forward for the professions. However, subsequent change in the focus of the NHS has resulted in the establishment of fewer posts than anticipated. Nevertheless, this position remains an aspiration for therapists and it has been suggested that they will attract experts and will take many years to achieve (Craik and McKay, 2003). However, as these posts require a balance of knowledge and skills in expert practice, leadership, education and research, therapists developing these may also be preparing for posts in academia, management or other arenas.

Maintaining a current CV

Keeping track of past and current experience has always been important, but with more varied employment patterns, it will be essential. However, it should be more that just a note of achievements. It will be important to look beyond the obvious to identify transferable skills that will be relevant in other contexts. As a review of expertise and knowledge obtained, it can become the basis for identifying areas for development. But it must be kept up to date, ready to be used.

Continuing professional development

Continuing professional development has been advocated by the College of Occupational Therapists and the Chartered Society of Physiotherapy for many years. However, the creation of the Health Professions Council and its requirement that evidence of continuing competence was needed to maintain registration has been a further impetus to its widespread adoption in the UK. The Health Professions Council (2006) requires that therapists have a written portfolio of their CPD, including varied activities relevant to current or future practice. Supervising students on practice placements is an excellent method of continuing professional development. This may be especially relevant for therapists working in a non-traditional or generic setting where providing a placement for a therapy student will not only retain contact with the profession but also contribute to the education of future therapists in these settings.

There is a need to show how the CPD has contributed to the quality of practice, service delivery and service users (Health Professions Council, 2006). Every 2 years, therapists have to confirm that they have maintained their continuing professional development and a small percentage of therapists will be audited. If registration lapses after a break in practice, additional measures will be needed to return to practice. Thus documenting activities and their relevance to practice will be necessary. The HPC suggests acceptable activities, including: work-based learning such as secondments or project work; professional activity such as mentoring or research supervision; self-directed learning such as reading articles or book reviews; other activities such as voluntary work and formal education (Health Professions Council, 2006).

Postgraduate study

There is a growing acceptance that in the rapidly changing work of health and social care, further training and education will be needed to provide recognition of additional knowledge and skills. This may take the form of short courses developing skills or study days about a specific clinical topic. For many therapists undertaking a practice educator or clinical supervisor course will be a key education activity. Increasingly therapists are interested in obtaining formal recognition for their study and there are many taught postgraduate courses which provide Postgraduate Certificate, Diploma and Master's level qualifications. Many can be studied on a part-time basis and there are also options of studying one or two modules before the need to register for a full qualification. While many of these are profession specific, others are designed for a more diverse audience.

Careful consideration will be required to choose the most relevant programme, and maintaining a professional focus will be important to make the link with continuing registration with the Health Professions Council. So a therapist in a clearly defined therapy post may seek a course to extend knowledge and skills in a wider direction, whereas someone in a generic or non-therapy post may find studying an MSc occupational therapy or MSc physiotherapy sustains an important professional connection that will be valuable when moving back into a more mainstream post.

Academic careers

For therapists wishing to pursue an academic career, postgraduate study will be essential. While some universities may consider applications from therapists with a Master's degree, a PhD will be needed in the future as will evidence of academic publications. Before pursuing this option, therapists may wish to obtain some lecturing experience and lecturer/practitioner posts are one way of doing this. Often this starts as a secondment, with therapists retaining their clinical post but being seconded to a university for a fixed time, often on a part-time basis. Although few therapists currently have a career exclusively in research, this option is likely to increase in the future.

Private practice

Although many people dream of the freedom of working for themselves, the reality is often very different. Working in private practice is usually an option for experienced therapists and not for novices. Working with an established practice, perhaps on a sessional or part-time basis while continuing with anther job, is a familiar route into this sector. For those who wish to establish their own private practice, business knowledge is required along with entrepreneurial skills, enhanced insurance cover and careful thought and advice. Both the Chartered Society of Physiotherapy and the College of Occupational Therapists offer guidance.

Conclusion

For current and future graduates, career planning is not as predictable as before. There will be threats but also many opportunities and how individual therapists perceive them will vary. Occupational therapy and physiotherapy pre-registration education is an excellent foundation not only for professional life but also for a wider sphere of activities. Maintaining a professional focus will be essential, and joining, and being an active member of, the relevant professional organisation will provide valuable advice. Registering, and maintaining registration, with the Health Professions Council through continuing professional development will be another strand in keeping that professional focus. The future will demand that therapists retain their key philosophies and principles but know how and when to be flexible and adaptable to meet changing circumstances. It would be a sad irony if therapists cannot respond to that challenge: one we so often expect in our clients.

References

Anon (2007) Breaking Out: Frontline 4 April 2007 http://www.csp.org.uk/director/newsandevents/frontline/archiveissues.cfm?ITEM_ID=B695E31E043D7589C6260EFC3531B496&article=#going (Accessed 6th November 2007).

Chartered Society of Physiotherapy (2003) *The New Chartered Physiotherapist: Guidelines of Good Practice for New Entrant to Physiotherapy*. London: Chartered Society of Physiotherapy.

Chartered Society of Physiotherapy (2006) *Guidance on Developing Student Placements in Community and Other Non-Traditional Settings*. London: Chartered Society of Physiotherapy.

College of Occupational Therapists (2004) *The Dr Elizabeth Casson Memorial Lectures 1973–2000*. London: College of Occupational Therapists.

College of Occupational Therapists (2002) *From interface to integration*. http://www.cot.co.uk/members/integration/pdf/strategy.pdf (Accessed 6th November 2007)

Craik, C. (2002) Basic solutions to the OT shortage? *Therapy Weekly*, 14th November.

Craik, C., McKay, E. (2003) Consultant therapists: recognising and developing expertise. Opinion Piece. *British Journal of Occupational Therapy* **66**(6), 281–283.

Craik, C. (2006) More graduates – opportunity or threat? *Occupational Therapy News* **14**(1), 22.

Department of Health (2000a) *The NHS Plan*. London: Stationery Office.

Department of Health (2000b) *Meeting the Challenge: a Strategy for the Allied Health Professions*. London: Department of Health.

Department of Health (2004) *The NHS Knowledge and Skills Framework and the Development Review Process*. London: Department of Health.

Department of Health (2006) *No excuses. Embrace partnership now. Step towards change!* Report of the third sector commissioning task force http://www.dh.gov.uk/en/Publicationsandstatistics/Publications/PublicationsPolicyAndGuidance/DH_4137144 (Accessed 3rd November 2007).

Department of Health (2007) *Social Partnership Forum Action Plan for Maximising Employment Opportunities for Newly Qualified Healthcare Professionals in a Changing NHS*. London: Department of Health.

Health Care Workforce (2005) http://www.healthcareworkforce.org.uk/C4/2005/Project%20Documentation/2006-07%20Summary%20WRT%20Recommendations.doc (Accessed 22nd November 2005).

Health Professions Council (2006) Continuing professional development and your registration, http://www.hpc-uk.org/assets/documents/10001314CPD_and_your_registration.pdf (Accessed 29th October 2007).

Henderson, S.E., Maciver, D. (2003) To PhD or not to PhD: the question is, where do we work? *British Journal of Occupational Therapy* **66**(10), 482–484.

Hobden, J. (2007) The global village. Frontline 04 July 2007 http://www.csp.org.uk/director/newsandevents/frontline/archiveissues.cfm?item_id=879964E0A845A94485A03FA5AD2BF2C6 (Accessed 6th November 2007).

NHS London (2007) *Healthcare for London: A Framework for Action*. http://www.healthcareforlondon.nhs.uk/pdf/aFrameworkForAction.pdf

Totten, C., Pratt, J. (2001) Innovation in fieldwork education: working with member of the homeless population in Glasgow. *British Journal of Occupational Therapy* **64**(11), 559–563.

Voluntary Service Overseas (2007) *Therapists and VSO* http://www.vso.org.uk/volunteering/therapists.asp (Accessed 28th October 2007).

Voluntary Service Overseas (2007) Youth for Development http://www.vso.org.uk/volunteering/youth/yfd/index.asp#0 (Accessed 28th October 2007).

Wood, A. (2005) Student practice contexts: changing face, changing place. *British Journal of Occupational Therapy* **68**(8), 375–378.

Professional and statutory bodies – documentation, standards and guidelines

Chartered Society of Physiotherapy (CSP) (2002) *General Principles of Record Keeping and Access to Health Records*. London: CSP.

Chartered Society of Physiotherapy (CSP) (2005) *Core Standards of Physiotherapy Practice*. London: CSP.

Chartered Society of Physiotherapy (CSP) (2005) *Service Standards of Physiotherapy Practice*. London: CSP.

College of Occupational Therapists (COT) (2006) *Record Keeping*. College of Occupational Therapists guidance 2. London: COT.

College of Occupational Therapists (2007) *Professional Standards for Occupational Therapy Practice*, 2nd edn. London: COT.

Council of Occupational Therapists of the European Countries (COTEC) (1996) *Code of Ethics and Standard of Practice*. London: COTEC.

General Social Care Council (GSCC) (2002) *Codes of Practice for Social Care Workers and Employers*. London: GSCC.

Health Professions Council (HPC) (2007) *Standards of Conduct, Performance and Ethics*. London: HPC.

Health Professions Council (HPC) (2007) *Standards of Proficiency*. London: HPC. (For each of 13 health professions regulated by the HPC.)

Nursing and Midwifery Council (NMC) (2007) *Record Keeping Guidance*. London: NMC.

Royal College of Physicians (RCP) (2007) *Setting Clinical Standards: Record Keeping Standards*. London: RCP.

World Confederation for Physical Therapy (WCPT) (2007) *Position Statements: Standards of Physical Therapy Practice*.

Resources for evidence-based practice

Centre for Evidence-Based Medicine
http://www.cebm.net/index.asp
Tools for learning how to practice and evaluate evidence-based medicine

Centre for Health Evidence
http://www.cche.net/usersguides/main.asp
Users' guides to evidence-based practice

National Electronic Library for Health
http://www.nelh.nhs.uk/
A range of resources to help healthcare decision-makers.

Database of Abstracts of Reviews of Effects (DARE)
http://www.york.ac.uk/inst/crd/darehp.htm
Research-based information about the effects of interventions used in health and social care.

Cochrane Collaboration of Systematic Reviews
http://www.cochrane.org/index0.htm
Up-to-date information about the effects of health care including systematic reviews.

Evidence-Based Clinical Knowledge Database – PRODIGY
http://www.prodigy.nhs.uk/
Evidence-based clinical knowledge on common conditions and symptoms managed by primary healthcare professionals.

NHS Health Development Agency
http://www.had-online.org.uk/
Evidence for policy makers, professionals and practitioners on what works to improve people's health and reduce health inequalities.

Bandolier
http://www.jr2.ox.ac.uk/bandolier/
Newsletter summarising the latest research on the effectiveness of health care interventions. Monthly.

Effective Health Care
http://www.york.ac.uk/inst/crd/ehcb.htm
Reports effectiveness of health care interventions based on systematic reviews and research synthesis. Bi-monthly.

Effectiveness Matters
http://www.york.ac.uk/inst/crd/em.htm
Updates on the effectiveness of important health interventions for practitioners and decision makers in the NHS. Linked to above.

Journal of Clinical Excellence
http://www.radcliffe-oxford.com/journals/
Evidence-based practice, clinical effectiveness, guidelines and clinical audit. Quarterly.

TRIP Database
http://www.tripdatabase.com/
Hyperlinked access to the largest collection of 'evidence-based' material on the web.

Centre for Evidence-Based Physiotherapy
http://www.cebp.nl/
Search, collect and disseminate available scientific evidence in the physiotherapy domain

PEDRO
http://www.pedro.fhs.usyd.edu.au/
Physiotherapy evidence database. Abstracts of randomised controlled trials, systematic reviews and evidence-based clinical practice guidelines. Most trials are quality rated.

Otseeker
http://www.otseeker.com/
Abstracts of systematic reviews and randomised controlled trials relevant to occupational therapy. Most trials are quality rated.

Occupational Therapy Evidence Based Practice Research Group
http://www-fhs.mcmaster.ca/rehab/ebp
Critical reviews of evidence regarding the effectiveness of occupational therapy interventions. Critical appraisal tools.

Index

Page numbers in *italics* represent figures, those in **bold** represent tables.